# Companion Workbook to Ways to Quit Drinking

A Sober Curious Book on How to Control Alcohol for Better Health, Self-Esteem and Mental Clarity

Michelle Matthews and Tony Matthews

# © Copyright 2024 - All rights reserved.

The content contained within this book may not be reproduced, duplicated or transmitted without direct written permission from the author or the publisher.

Under no circumstances will any blame or legal responsibility be held against the publisher, or author, for any damages, reparation, or monetary loss due to the information contained within this book, either directly or indirectly.

Legal Notice:

This book is copyright protected. It is only for personal use. You cannot amend, distribute, sell, use, quote or paraphrase any part, or the content within this book, without the consent of the author or publisher.

Disclaimer Notice:

Please note the information contained within this document is for educational and entertainment purposes only. All effort has been executed to present accurate, up to date, reliable, complete information. No warranties of any kind are declared or implied. Readers acknowledge that the author is not engaged in the rendering of legal, financial, medical or professional advice. The content within this book has been derived from various sources. Please consult a licensed professional before attempting any techniques outlined in this book.

By reading this document, the reader agrees that under no circumstances is the author responsible for any losses, direct or indirect, that are incurred as a result of the use of the information contained within this document, including, but not limited to, errors, omissions, or inaccuracies.

# Table of Contents

IN GOOD COMPANY ........................................................................................................... 1
    OBSERVATION AND REFLECTION ................................................................................. 4

WELCOME .......................................................................................................................... 5

CHAPTER 1: IN THE BEGINNING THERE WAS WATER... AND THEN ALONG CAME ALCOHOL –
APPLYING IT TO YOUR LIFE ................................................................................................ 7
    OVERVIEW ................................................................................................................... 7
    READING ASSIGNMENT, CHAPTER 1 ........................................................................... 8
    SUMMARY POINTS FROM CHAPTER 1 OF WAYS TO QUIT DRINKING ......................... 8
    PURPOSE OF WORKBOOK CHAPTER 1 ....................................................................... 9
    EXERCISES FOR CHAPTER 1 ........................................................................................ 9
        *Fill in the Blanks – Industrial Applications* ........................................................ 9
        *Multiple Choice Quiz – Lesser-Known Health Impacts* ................................... 10
        *Self-Reflection Questions – Awareness of Alcohol and Its Effects* ................ 13
        *Notes* ............................................................................................................... 14

CHAPTER 2: WHY DO PEOPLE DEVELOP ISSUES WITH ALCOHOL? – APPLYING IT TO YOUR LIFE .. 17
    OVERVIEW ................................................................................................................. 17
    READING ASSIGNMENT, CHAPTER 2 ......................................................................... 18
    SUMMARY POINTS FROM CHAPTER 2 OF WAYS TO QUIT DRINKING ....................... 19
    PURPOSE OF WORKBOOK CHAPTER 2 ..................................................................... 20
    EXERCISES FOR CHAPTER 2 ...................................................................................... 21
        *Which Ones Can You Relate to Being Influenced By? – External Factors* ..... 21
        *Which Ones Can You Relate to Being Influenced By? – Internal Factors* ...... 22
        *What Is Your Suspicion?* ................................................................................. 23
        *Self-Reflection Questions – Contributing Factors* .......................................... 24
        *Notes* ............................................................................................................... 25

CHAPTER 3: YOUR 'WHY' FOR QUITTING DRINKING – APPLYING IT TO YOUR LIFE ............. 27
    OVERVIEW ................................................................................................................. 27
    READING ASSIGNMENT, CHAPTER 3 ......................................................................... 28
        *Something to Understand About 'Working Out What We Want'* .................. 28
    SUMMARY POINTS FROM CHAPTER 3 OF WAYS TO QUIT DRINKING ....................... 29
    PURPOSE OF WORKBOOK CHAPTER 3 ..................................................................... 30
    EXERCISES FOR CHAPTER 3 ...................................................................................... 31
        *Exercise 1: Reflecting on Your Personal 'Why'* ............................................... 31
        *Exercise 2: Visualisation and Future Pacing* ................................................... 35
        *Summary of the Two Exercises* ....................................................................... 39
        *Notes* ............................................................................................................... 40

CHAPTER 4: BREAKING FREE FROM ALCOHOL – A PRACTICAL LOOK AT WAYS TO STOP DRINKING
– APPLYING IT TO YOUR LIFE ........................................................................................... 43

- Overview ........................................................................................................ 43
- Reading Assignment, Chapter 4 .................................................................. 44
- Summary Points From Chapter 4 of *Ways to Quit Drinking* ........................ 44
- Purpose of Workbook Chapter 4 .................................................................. 57
- Exercise for Chapter 4 .................................................................................. 58
  - Exercise 1: Which Option Will You Adopt? ............................................ 58
  - Notes ...................................................................................................... 59

## CHAPTER 5: WHEN YOU KNOW YOU NEED TO STOP DRINKING – APPLYING IT TO YOUR LIFE .... 61

- Overview ........................................................................................................ 61
  - Step 1: Realisation That There Is a Problem ......................................... 61
  - Step 2: Information Gathering, Decision Time and Action Time ........... 61
  - Step 3: Managing the Decision Long-Term ........................................... 62
- Reading Assignment, Chapter 5 .................................................................. 62
- Summary Points from Chapter 5 of *Ways to Quit Drinking* ........................ 62
- Purpose of Workbook Chapter 5 .................................................................. 63
- Exercises for Chapter 5 ................................................................................ 64
  - Step 1: Realisation That There Is a Problem ......................................... 64
  - Step 2: Information Gathering, Decision Time and Action Time ........... 75
  - Step 3: Managing the Decision Long-Term ........................................... 75
  - Notes ...................................................................................................... 78

## CHAPTER 6: PUTTING IT INTO PRACTICE – APPLYING IT TO YOUR LIFE ........................... 81

- Overview ........................................................................................................ 81
  - Why This Chapter Matters ..................................................................... 81
- Reading Assignment, Chapter 6 .................................................................. 81
- Summary Points from Chapter 6 of *Ways to Quit Drinking* ........................ 82
- Purpose of Workbook Chapter 6 .................................................................. 83
- Exercises for Chapter 6 ................................................................................ 84
  - Exercise 1: Action Plan – Template One ............................................... 84
  - Exercise 2: Action Plan – Template Two ............................................... 93
- Keys to Success ............................................................................................ 95
  - Notes ...................................................................................................... 95

## WRAP-UP: YOUR JOURNEY TOWARDS BETTER HEALTH, SELF-ESTEEM AND MENTAL CLARITY ... 99

- Embracing Your Exciting Future ................................................................... 99
- Nurturing Self-Care and Healing .................................................................. 99
- Celebrating Your Progress ......................................................................... 100
- Looking Ahead ............................................................................................ 100
- Final Thoughts ............................................................................................ 100

## APPENDIX .................................................................................................... 101

- Fill in the Blanks – Industrial Applications ................................................. 101
- Multiple Choice Quiz – Lesser-Known Health Impacts ............................. 101

## REFERENCES ............................................................................................... 103

# In Good Company

If you choose to abstain from drinking alcohol, you're in good company. Like-minded people (who you might imagine possess the means to have and do whatever they jolly well please) include:

- **Bradley Cooper:** An American actor and filmmaker known for his roles in films like *Silver Linings Playbook*, *American Sniper* and *A Star is Born*.

- **Blake Lively:** An American actress famous for her role in the TV series *Gossip Girl* and movies like *The Age of Adaline* and *A Simple Favor*.

- **Daniel Radcliffe:** A British actor best known for playing Harry Potter in the *Harry Potter* film series.

- **Kristin Davis:** An American actress best known for her role as Charlotte York in the TV series *Sex and the City*.

- **Eminem:** An American rapper, songwriter and record producer known for hits like *Lose Yourself*, *Not Afraid* and *Love the Way You Lie*.

- **Jennifer Lopez:** An American singer, actress and dancer known for her music hits like *Jenny from the Block* and movies like *Selena* and *Hustlers*.

- **Tyler, the Creator:** An American rapper, singer and record producer known for his albums like *IGOR* and *Flower Boy*.

- **Pharrell Williams:** An American singer, rapper, songwriter and record producer known for hits like *Happy* and his work with the production duo The Neptunes.

- **Naomi Campbell:** A British supermodel and actress known for her work in the fashion industry and appearances on TV shows like *The Face*.

- **Zendaya:** An American actress and singer known for her roles in the TV series *Euphoria* and the *Spider-Man* films

- **Jennifer Hudson:** An American singer and actress, winner of an Academy Award for her role in *Dreamgirls* and a finalist on *American Idol*.

- **Gerard Butler:** A Scottish actor known for his roles in films like *300*, *P.S. I Love You* and *Olympus Has Fallen*.

- **Kim Cattrall:** A British Canadian actress best known for her role as Samantha Jones in the TV series *Sex and the City*.

- **Calvin Harris:** A Scottish DJ, record producer and singer known for hits like *Feel So Close* and *Summer*.

- **Lucy Hale:** An American actress and singer known for her role in the TV series *Pretty Little Liars*.

- **Tim McGraw:** An American country singer and actor known for hits like *Live Like You Were Dying* and his role in the movie *The Blind Side*.

- **Lana Del Rey:** An American singer and songwriter known for her albums like *Born to Die* and *Norman F**ing Rockwell!*

- **Cristiano Ronaldo:** A Portuguese professional footballer, often regarded as one of the greatest football players of all time.

- **Warren Buffett:** An American business magnate, investor and philanthropist who is chairman and CEO of Berkshire Hathaway.

- **Rafael Nadal:** A Spanish professional tennis player, considered one of the greatest tennis players in history.

- **Mike Pence:** An American politician who served as the 48th Vice President of the United States.

- **Mitt Romney:** An American politician and businessman, serving as the junior United States senator from Utah.

- **Moby:** An American musician, songwriter and producer known for his electronic music and vegan activism.

- **Lewis Hamilton:** A British Formula 1 driver for Mercedes, regarded as one of the greatest F1 drivers of all time with multiple world championship titles.

- **Tony Kanaan:** A Brazilian racing driver who has competed in the IndyCar Series and won the 2013 Indianapolis 500.

- **Brené Brown:** An American research professor, lecturer, author and podcast host known for her work on vulnerability, courage, shame and empathy. She has written several bestselling books, including *Daring Greatly* and *Braving the Wilderness*.

- **Jamie Lee Curtis:** An American actress and author known for her roles in films such as *Halloween, True Lies* and *Freaky Friday*. She is also an advocate for recovery from addiction and has been open about her journey with sobriety.

- **Eva Mendes:** An American actress, model and businesswoman known for her roles in films like *Hitch* and *The Place Beyond the Pines*.

- **Joe Manganiello:** An American actor known for his roles in *True Blood* and *Magic Mike*.

- **Colin Farrell:** An Irish actor known for his roles in films such as *In Bruges, The Lobster* and *Phone Booth*. He has been open about his sobriety and past struggles with addiction.

- **Robert Downey Jr.:** An American actor best known for his role as Iron Man in the Marvel Cinematic Universe. He has been sober since 2003 after overcoming a highly publicised struggle with addiction.

- **Elton John:** A British singer, pianist and composer known for his hit songs like *Rocket Man, Tiny Dancer* and *Your Song*. He has been sober since 1990.

- **Tyra Banks:** An American television personality, model, producer and businesswoman known for creating and hosting *America's Next Top Model*.

- **Keith Urban:** A New Zealand Australian country music singer, songwriter and guitarist. He has been open about his recovery from addiction and has maintained his sobriety since 2006.

- **Tom Hardy:** A British actor known for his roles in films like *Inception, The Dark Knight Rises* and *Mad Max: Fury Road*. He has been open about his decision to quit alcohol to maintain a healthier lifestyle.

According to publicly available information, these people in the public eye have chosen to abstain from drinking alcohol. Whether they never drank in the past or have more recently chosen abstinence for optimal health or to address issues with alcohol, it matters little. What's significant is the message their choices convey.

# Observation and Reflection

What are your thoughts on the fact that so many people who are highly successful in their chosen fields choose not to drink alcohol?

_____
_____
_____
_____
_____
_____
_____
_____
_____
_____
_____
_____

Athletes like Cristiano Ronaldo attribute their physical fitness in part to their non-drinking habits. Musician Ed Sheeran addressed his over-drinking habit, reined it in and found it beneficial for his creativity. Actor Bradley Cooper has been alcohol free for almost two decades, helping him focus on his career. These individuals, as well as many others, are a testament that you can lead an exciting, successful life without relying on alcohol.

Choosing to be alcohol free offers immense power and conscious choice. When your decisions align with a goal of better health and mental clarity, you wake up energised, focused and with a sense of purpose you wouldn't get if you were prioritising the temporary relief provided by alcohol. Remember, choosing not to drink doesn't make you boring or uncool. Instead, it puts you in an elite group of people who prioritise their wellbeing above societal norms.

So, if someone offers you a drink at a party, remember – saying no doesn't mean missing out, but rather making a conscious choice towards a healthier and more fulfilling lifestyle.

# Welcome

Dear reader,

Welcome to the official Companion Workbook for *Ways to Quit Drinking*. We are thrilled that you have decided to take this significant step towards a healthier and more fulfilling life! This Companion Workbook is designed to accompany you on your way forward, providing practical exercises, insights and reflections that will help you apply the knowledge from the main book in meaningful and helpful ways.

As you travel on this path, it's essential to remember that knowledge is power – but that the *application* of that knowledge is where true transformation occurs. Reading widely and consuming as much information as possible (and as you can cope with!) on this topic will be invaluable. Sometimes, it takes hearing the same message from different sources or at different times for it to crystallise clearly in our minds. So, don't ever give up. Keep making incremental improvements and know that every step forward is a step towards something better for you, as well as for those who love you.

Our own unhealthy relationships with alcohol began pretty much like anyone else's might have. As a couple in our 40s living in the suburbs, on the surface we seemed to have a normal family life. And on most fronts, it was (and still is) brilliant! However, behind closed doors, we were struggling silently with drinking more than we knew was wise. What started as a way to unwind and socialise in our 20s gradually became a dependence on daily 'drinkies time' that impacted our health, self-esteem, productivity, relationship and overall wellbeing.

Personally (Michelle), for over a decade I grappled with the consequences of my drinking habits, vocalising to Tony my self-disapproval and explaining my ineffectual and sometimes comical methods to abstain (eating pickled onions doesn't work!). While I continued to function 'normally', my mornings were often spent with a pounding head and stinging eyes from the previous night's indulgence. Daily vows to 'not do that again' invariably failed by mid-afternoon, and the shame and frustration grew and grew. It wasn't until a moment of sheer frustration that I decided to quit drinking for 12 months. The relief and elation I felt after just three weeks of being alcohol free were so profound that I then chose to live alcohol free permanently. Observing this (and with his own thoughts, struggles and observations held within), Tony joined me. Over time, we together crafted a plan to maintain our alcohol-free lifestyle.

We understand on an intimate level the struggle to control alcohol – because we've been there: not being honest with ourselves about how much (over the recommended limits) we were drinking, feeling the associated weight of shame and trying countless times to cut back, without much success. Not for very long, anyway. But – determined not to destroy our health for the future, nor to continue to show our children a way we did not want them to live – we found a way out, and we are passionate about sharing our insights with you.

This Companion Workbook will provide you with a way to closely examine the tools and strategies we used to overcome our dependence on alcohol. From understanding why problem drinking develops to exploring various options for quitting and outlining a step-by-step process for lasting change, we cover it all. We combine scientific rigour with personal experience to offer you a compassionate and evidence-based approach.

Consider us your neighbours who have walked a similar path. We won't pretend to have all the answers, but we will guide you compassionately towards your own path forward. We hope that within these pages, you will find gold nuggets of wisdom that help clear your path and enable you to achieve your goals.

Remember, healing and happiness await you beyond the shadows of alcohol dependence. Progress won't necessarily be easy, but with persistence and dedication, you can transform your life. We are honoured to accompany you on this path and excited to see the positive changes you will create.

Thank you for allowing us to be a part of your journey. We wish you strength, clarity and unwavering determination as you move forward.

Warmest regards,

Michelle and Tony

xo

# Chapter 1:

# In the Beginning There Was Water… And Then Along Came Alcohol – Applying It to Your Life

## Overview

Welcome to the first chapter of your Companion Workbook to *Ways to Quit Drinking*, where we dive into the complex world of alcohol. In the main book, Chapter 1 explores the dual nature of alcohol as both a social lubricant and a potential source of health issues. Now, in this Companion Workbook, our goal is to delve deeper into each facet of alcohol's influence on our lives, helping you to understand its place in your own journey.

If you don't already, you'll soon come to understand how alcohol is deeply woven into the fabric of society, offering both benefits and risks. From its ancient origins as a social and ritualistic beverage to its current role in global economics and healthcare systems, alcohol's impact is undeniable. Chapter 1 examines the origins of alcohol, its diverse industrial applications and its cultural significance. We will also highlight the pros and cons of alcohol consumption, from its potential health benefits to the risks of addiction, health issues and societal costs.

Our aim here is not to preach against alcohol, nor to glorify it. Instead, we will provide you with a balanced perspective, equipping you with the knowledge to make informed decisions about the role of alcohol in your own life. By understanding both the benefits and the downsides, you can navigate the complexities of the consequences of alcohol consumption with clarity and confidence.

Let's begin our exploration into the world of alcohol, understanding its historical, cultural and scientific dimensions and reflecting on how it impacts our lives today. This will help empower you to make choices that align with your personal values and goals.

# Reading Assignment, Chapter 1

Read Chapter 1 of *Ways to Quit Drinking: A Sober Curious Book on How to Control Alcohol for Better Health, Self-Esteem and Mental Clarity*. Take notes on anything that you did not previously know about, that surprised you, that alarmed you or simply that you thought was noteworthy or interesting. You may also like to make a note of one or two things that you'd like to research more closely at a later time. Curiosity is good. Asking questions is excellent.

_____
_____
_____
_____
_____
_____
_____
_____
_____

# Summary Points From Chapter 1 of *Ways to Quit Drinking*

- Alcohol is a double-edged sword, offering social and health benefits like relaxation and (some claim) heart health benefits (e.g., red wine), but also causing numerous health problems and societal issues when consumed excessively.

- It plays a significant role in social interactions, acting as an icebreaker and social lubricant, but can lead to impaired judgement and reckless decisions.

- Economically, alcohol contributes to job creation and tax revenues, yet incurs costs related to healthcare, law enforcement and lost productivity due to alcohol-related illnesses and accidents.

- Historically, alcohol has been intertwined with human civilisation since ancient times, serving roles in religion, medicine and social customs and evolving alongside advances in fermentation and distillation.

- The chapter examines both the pros and cons of alcohol objectively, providing insights into its benefits and harms to empower informed decision-making about personal consumption.

# Purpose of Workbook Chapter 1

When you have finished with Workbook Chapter 1, you will:

- Understand the dual nature of alcohol, recognising its benefits when consumed in moderation and its potential harms when consumed excessively.

- Recognise the social and cultural roles of alcohol in different societies and how these influence personal and social behaviours.

- Be aware of the economic impact of alcohol consumption, both positive and negative, on society and individuals.

- Appreciate the historical significance of alcohol, its evolution and its changing role in human civilisations over time.

- Have developed a balanced perspective on alcohol, enabling informed decision-making about your personal consumption based on a deeper understanding of its impacts.

These points provide a clear understanding of the main themes discussed in Chapter 1 of *Ways to Quit Drinking*, empowering you to reflect on your own attitudes and behaviours towards alcohol.

# Exercises for Chapter 1

For the answers to the questions in each exercise, please see the Appendix at the end of the book.

## *Fill in the Blanks – Industrial Applications*

1. _____ and _____ are types of alcohol that are commonly used as disinfectants because of their germ-killing properties.

2. Alcohol is used in the _____ of organisms, from microbes to cells, enabling scientific advances.

3. Ethanol and methanol can be used for de-icing planes and vehicle windshields because they have a lower _____ point than water.

4. When ethanol is blended into fuel, it burns more cleanly than gasoline, thus reducing dependence on _____ fuels.

5. The unique chemical properties of the _____ form of alcohol (_____ is what we consume as 'drinking alcohol') have proven invaluable over centuries of human innovation. We have only just begun to tap into alcohol's potential (e.g., its use as a biofuel) to advance progress.

## *Multiple Choice Quiz – Lesser-Known Health Impacts*

1. Which organisation classified alcoholic beverages as a Group 1 carcinogen?

    A. American Cancer Society (ACS)

    B. Centers for Disease Control and Prevention (CDC)

    C. International Agency for Research on Cancer (IARC)

    D. National Institutes of Health (NIH)

2. What is the relationship between alcohol consumption and breast cancer risk?

    A. Alcohol consumption decreases breast cancer risk.

    B. Alcohol consumption has no effect on breast cancer risk.

    C. Alcohol consumption increases breast cancer risk.

    D. The relationship between alcohol and breast cancer is inconclusive.

3. Besides breast cancer, alcohol consumption has been linked to an increased risk of which of the following cancers?

    A. Prostate cancer

    B. Pancreatic cancer

    C. Thyroid cancer

    D. Skin cancer

4. Which health issue is directly caused by excessive alcohol consumption?

    A. Type 2 diabetes

    B. Osteoporosis

    C. Liver disease

    D. Asthma

5. How does heavy drinking affect heart health?

    A. It reduces blood pressure.

    B. It improves heart rhythm.

    C. It can elevate blood pressure and disrupt heart rhythm.

    D. It has no effect on heart health.

6. Which statement about alcohol and brain health is true?

    A. Alcohol consumption reduces the risk of Alzheimer's disease.

    B. Alcohol has no impact on cognitive function.

    C. Chronic heavy drinking can lead to cognitive impairment and memory loss.

    D. Alcohol consumption improves memory and cognitive function.

7. Which oral health issue is associated with alcohol consumption?

    A. Sinus infections

    B. Tooth decay

    C. Hair loss

    D. Broken bones

8. How does alcohol consumption contribute to bad breath?

    A. By increasing saliva production.

    B. By neutralising acids in the mouth.

C. By drying out the mouth and promoting bacterial growth.

D. By strengthening tooth enamel.

9. How does alcohol consumption affect REM sleep?

    A. It enhances REM sleep duration and quality.

    B. It has no effect on REM sleep.

    C. It suppresses REM sleep.

    D. It increases the frequency of REM sleep.

10. What role does REM sleep play in memory and cognitive function?

    A. It has no impact on memory.

    B. It is essential for memory consolidation and learning.

    C. It only affects short-term memory.

    D. It primarily affects emotional memory.

11. How does alcohol consumption potentially increase the risk of Alzheimer's disease?

    A. By reducing blood pressure during sleep.

    B. By improving the quality of REM sleep.

    C. By disrupting the brain's process of clearing out harmful toxins.

    D. By decreasing the production of beta-amyloid proteins.

12. What risk is associated with moderate alcohol consumption during pregnancy?

    A. Increased intelligence in children

    B. Lower risk of preterm birth

    C. Higher risk of cognitive development issues

    D. Reduced likelihood of sudden infant death syndrome (SIDS).

13. What is the primary reason why alcohol consumption during pregnancy is discouraged?

    A. To promote weight gain in the baby.

    B. To reduce the risk of premature birth.

    C. To prevent cognitive impairments.

    D. To safeguard foetal health.

14. What is the main message conveyed about alcohol consumption in Chapter 1?

    A. Alcohol consumption should be avoided entirely.

    B. Mindful observation and consideration of alcohol's effects are encouraged.

    C. Alcohol advertisements and media portrayals should be ignored.

    D. Alcohol consumption is harmless and beneficial.

15. As a takeaway from Chapter 1, why is it suggested that it's important to observe alcohol mindfully in daily life?

    A. To notice how much alcohol others consume.

    B. To contemplate the effects of alcohol on personal relationships.

    C. To understand how alcohol is portrayed in the media.

    D. To assess how alcohol affects you.

## *Self-Reflection Questions – Awareness of Alcohol and Its Effects*

What are the main three facts you learned about alcohol as a result of reading Chapter 1: In the Beginning There Was Water… And Then Along Came Alcohol?

1. _____

2. _____

3. _____

Have any of the facts in this chapter changed the thoughts and feelings you have about your intake of alcohol? If yes, what has changed?

_____
_____
_____
_____
_____
_____
_____

Do you feel more informed and more knowledgeable about alcohol after reading this chapter? If yes, do you also feel more empowered to make decisions about the role alcohol has in your life?

_____
_____
_____
_____
_____
_____
_____

## Notes

_____
_____
_____
_____
_____
_____
_____
_____

# Chapter 2:

# Why Do People Develop Issues With Alcohol? – Applying It to Your Life

## Overview

In this chapter of the Companion Workbook, we will explore the wide variety of factors behind the development of problematic relationships with alcohol. This exploration involves delving into both external and internal factors that shape how a person interacts with alcohol. By understanding these influences, we can gain a much better view of the challenges we face and the steps necessary to overcome them.

The chapter therefore provides a clear and structured examination of environmental, social and cultural influences (external factors) as well as genetic, biological, psychological and personality influences (internal factors). Recognising the intricate web of these influences is crucial: It helps us understand that problematic alcohol use is not merely a matter of willpower and is certainly not a moral failing, but rather the result of a complex interplay of various elements.

By examining external factors, such as societal norms, accessibility, peer pressure and advertising, we uncover the powerful impact of our environment on our drinking behaviours. Similarly, by investigating internal factors, such as genetic predispositions, brain chemistry, mental health conditions and personality traits, we acknowledge the deep-rooted personal vulnerabilities that contribute to alcohol dependence.

This chapter is designed to equip you with knowledge and insights, fostering a compassionate understanding of your own very personal and individual relationship with alcohol. By gaining clarity on these factors, you will be better prepared to develop effective strategies for breaking free from the grip of alcohol and moving towards a healthier, more fulfilling life.

Is there anything more exciting than paving the way for empowerment and positive change?

# Reading Assignment, Chapter 2

As you read Chapter 2 of *Ways to Quit Drinking: A Sober Curious Book on How to Control Alcohol for Better Health, Self-Esteem and Mental Clarity*, focus on the external and internal factors described. Reflect on the following questions and prompts:

- **External factors:**

    o Contemplate the external factors discussed in this chapter. Do any of them resonate with you? Which ones have you personally experienced?

    o Did you realise you were affected by these factors before they were explicitly pointed out here?

    o Have you noticed any other external factors influencing your relationship with alcohol that haven't been covered in this chapter?

- **Internal factors:**

    o Consider the internal factors described. Do they make sense to you? Do any resonate with your experiences?

    o Do you think any of these internal factors might be playing a part in your relationship with alcohol?

- Make a note of your thoughts and feelings about these internal and external factors that influence our individual relationships with alcohol. What insights have you gained? How do you feel about these influences?

Take notes as you read to clarify your thoughts and deepen your understanding. Try to enjoy this exploration, because learning and growing as a person is fulfilling and what life is all about. But do be aware that some of the realisations that come to you as a result of what is pointed out here might stir up emotions like sadness, frustration, regret, disappointment and even anger. These emotions are important. Observe what comes up and take notes for future reference. In general, it's important to acknowledge and address emotions, because sometimes *not* addressing them can cause us big problems.

_____

_____

_____

_____

# Summary Points From Chapter 2 of *Ways to Quit Drinking*

- **External factors:**

    o Social environment, including peer pressure and cultural norms, plays a significant role.

    o Stressful life events and coping mechanisms influence alcohol consumption.

    o Accessibility and availability of alcohol contribute to drinking habits.

    o Marketing and media portrayal affect perceptions and behaviours related to alcohol.

    o Family history and upbringing influence attitudes towards alcohol.

- **Internal factors:**

    o Genetic predisposition can increase susceptibility to alcohol dependence.

    o Psychological factors such as anxiety, depression and low self-esteem contribute to alcohol use.

    o Personal beliefs and expectations about alcohol's effects play a role.

    o Coping styles and personality traits influence how individuals manage stress and emotions with alcohol.

- **Intersection of internal and external factors:**

    o Both internal and external factors interact to shape an individual's relationship with alcohol.

    o Understanding these factors can help identify triggers and develop effective strategies for moderation or abstinence.

    o Awareness of these influences can empower individuals to make informed choices about their alcohol consumption.

- **Holistic approach to understanding alcohol use:**

    o Recognising the complexity of factors involved in alcohol use helps in developing a comprehensive approach to managing it.

    o Addressing both internal and external factors is crucial for sustainable behaviour change.

    o Self-reflection and awareness are key to understanding one's relationship with alcohol and making positive changes.

## Purpose of Workbook Chapter 2

When you have finished with Workbook Chapter 2, you will have:

- Identified which of the described external factors (social pressures, accessibility and cultural norms) surround you – now and in the past – and how they've likely influenced your personal relationship with alcohol.

- Understood how messages in the media impact your alcohol consumption habits.

- Recognised the role of family history and societal influences in shaping your views on drinking.

- Reflected on your own experiences with the various external factors and how they may have influenced your relationship with alcohol.

- Gained insights into the internal factors that contribute to your alcohol use, including genetics, psychological factors and personal beliefs.

- Contemplated how stress and anxiety, depression and coping mechanisms affect your relationship with alcohol.

- Evaluated your personality traits and coping styles in relation to alcohol use.

- Recognised the interaction between internal and external factors in shaping your individual relationship with alcohol.

- Begun to contemplate how you might develop strategies for managing these influences to begin making positive changes in your alcohol consumption habits.

# Exercises for Chapter 2

## *Which Ones Can You Relate to Being Influenced By? – External Factors*

Cast your eyes over the words below. Each one represents an external factor that may influence a person to think, feel or act in a certain way with regard to alcohol. If you recognise or identify that the factor has likely influenced your relationship with alcohol, circle it.

*Do you notice? Many of the words and phrases refer to essentially the same thing. Often, it takes seeing the same thing from a variety of perspectives before we can recognise it for what it is. This 'word cloud' is designed to stimulate your thinking and trigger memories to enable you to identify which factors have been instrumental in the development of your relationship with alcohol – and thus highlight where your attention may possibly need to be focused to overcome a detrimental relationship.*

| Branding | Parties | Workplace culture | Social pressures | Influential people |
|---|---|---|---|---|
| Easy access | Public attitudes | College life | Celebrations | Social media |
| Festivals | Drinking venues | Nightlife | Friends | Social drinking |
| Peer influence | Holidays | Marketing | Work environment | Availability |
| Affordable pricing | Social events | Cultural norms | Customs | Proximity |
| Social expectations | Legal availability (drinking age) | Accessibility | Social exposure | Economic factors |
| Acquaintances | Family dynamics | Romantic partners | Media messages | Drinking 'games' (e.g., beer pong) |
| Policies (e.g., alcohol stores in or next to supermarkets; alcohol home delivery services, etc.) | Community support | Advertising | Popularity | Social acceptance |

Have you realised that there are additional external factors that do not appear above that have influenced your relationship with alcohol? Below, make a note of any you think of:

_____
_____
_____
_____
_____
_____
_____

## Which Ones Can You Relate to Being Influenced By? – Internal Factors

Again, cast your eyes over the words below, each one representing an internal factor that may influence a person to think, feel or act in a certain way with regard to alcohol. If you recognise or identify that the factor has likely influenced your relationship with alcohol, circle it. Circle it many times if it is a very strong influence for you.

| Stress | Habit | Trauma/childhood trauma | Self-medication | Poor self-esteem |
|---|---|---|---|---|
| Genetic predisposition | Anxiety | (Lack of) Emotional regulation | Personality traits | Identity |
| Social confidence | Mental health disorders | Depression | Impulsivity | Boredom |
| Coping mechanisms | (Response to) Peer pressure | Emotional pain | Loneliness | Past experiences |
| Guilt | Fear | Shame | Anger | Unresolved conflict |
| Desire for escapism | Personal beliefs | (Response to) Cultural influences | Family history | Unmet needs |
| Absence of sense of belonging | Unclear personal values | Sub-par life satisfaction | Cognitive distortions | Genetic predisposition |
| Alcohol's effect on the brain (e.g., dopamine, relaxation) | Low emotional resilience | Sensation seeker | Limited social support systems | Unidentified or no sense of purpose |

Do you perceive additional internal factors that have influenced your relationship with alcohol? Below, make a note of any more you think of that are relevant:

_____
_____
_____
_____
_____
_____
_____

## *What Is Your Suspicion?*

If we were conducting a scientific experiment, we might now be proposing a hypothesis – our best guess about what external and internal factors unique to us have led to a relationship with alcohol that is not healthy, does not please us and is not fulfilling or conducive to a long and vibrant life.

We're not making any professional medical diagnoses here – and nor do we need to. It is sufficient to gain some basic clarity about the factors at play in order to relieve ourselves of the thought – and perhaps guilt – that we are somehow lacking in willpower or are of poor moral character.

### *Your Wellbeing, Your Passion Project*

Having said that, it's always a good idea to have a primary care provider to oversee our general physical and mental health – including aspects of our diet that may or may not serve us. Do be discerning in who you choose as your main healthcare provider (your overweight general practitioner who drinks too much themselves is unlikely to give you the balanced discussion you may be seeking). We're all for treating our physical and mental health like a passion project, seeking to master the underpinning fundamentals (sleep, diet, exercise, mindfulness, meditation… and so on) in order to win at this life game!

## *Self-Reflection Questions – Contributing Factors*

Write down the *top three factors* that you believe are the strongest *external* contributors to your current relationship with alcohol:

1. _____

2. _____

3. _____

Write down the *top three factors* that you believe are the strongest *internal* contributors to your current relationship with alcohol:

1. _____

2. _____

3. _____

Did any of the facts in this chapter change the thoughts and feelings you have about your intake of alcohol? If yes, what has changed?

_____

_____

_____

_____

_____

Do you feel more informed and more knowledgeable about alcohol after reading this chapter? If yes, do you also feel more empowered to make decisions about the role alcohol has in your life?

_____

_____

_____

_____

_____

_____

_____

## Notes

# Chapter 3:

# Your 'Why' for Quitting Drinking – Applying It to Your Life

## Overview

In Chapter 3, we delve into the crucial first step of any meaningful change: understanding your 'why'. This chapter invites you to deeply reflect on the core motivations that drive your desire to reassess and potentially alter your relationship with alcohol. Pinpointing these personal incentives is essential to maintaining your resolve when challenges arise.

The chapter explores four significant areas that might resonate with your motivations:

- **Health and longevity:** Reflect on how alcohol might be conflicting with your aspirations for a long, active and vibrant life.

- **Quality of life:** Consider whether alcohol is enhancing or detracting from your daily energy and overall wellbeing.

- **Positive role modeling:** Think about the example you're setting for young people and those who look up to you, and how your drinking habits might influence their future behaviours.

- **Nurturing relationships:** Examine how alcohol might be silently straining your close connections and affecting the quality of your interactions with loved ones.

By exploring these aspects, this chapter will help you uncover your unique reasons for considering a life with reduced or no alcohol. Your 'why' might encompass elements from the areas noted above or include other personal incentives that haven't been listed.

Chapter 3 builds on the factual groundwork laid in the first two chapters, encouraging insightful self-inquiry to reveal your distinctive motivations. Understanding why this exploration is important to you will provide the clarity and conviction necessary to stay committed to your goals.

We hope you do embrace this journey of self-discovery, as it lights the way towards a healthier, more fulfilling life.

# Reading Assignment, Chapter 3

Read Chapter 3 of Ways to Quit Drinking: A Sober Curious Book on How to Control Alcohol for Better Health, Self-Esteem and Mental Clarity.

Without attempting to 'force' any singular, meaningful answer (which can sometimes be the case when we're exploring something as all-encompassing and potentially life-changing as identifying our 'why'), make notes on anything that jumps out at you as you read through the chapter.

_____
_____
_____
_____
_____
_____

### *Something to Understand About 'Working Out What We Want'*

Scientific studies suggest that the process of self-reflection and introspection can significantly help a person understand what they truly want in life. This process involves quieting the mind, perhaps by engaging in mindfulness practices such as meditation or yoga, and by spending time in nature, such as walking among trees or at the beach.

According to a study published in the *Journal of Personality and Social Psychology*, people who engage in regular self-reflection are more likely to have a clearer understanding of their own values, passions and goals (Grant et al., 2002). They are also more likely to experience higher levels of happiness and satisfaction with their lives.

Another research study, from Stanford University, found that walking, especially in natural environments like a deserted beach or a forest trail, can boost creative thinking and problem-solving skills (Oppezzo & Schwartz, 2014). This can help you get back to your core desires, which you may have lost sight of due to daily life stressors and the bombardment of messages from society about what you 'should' want or be.

So, there is definitely immense power in taking some time for yourself to sit quietly with your thoughts.

When all your decisions come from a place of deep understanding about what you truly want (even if it means going against societal norms or expectations), you wake up motivated, with clarity and purpose.

This sense of direction is something you never get if you're constantly reacting to external pressures without taking the time to listen to your inner voice. So, if you don't do this already, it may pay to work out how you can take some time out for yourself – to regularly walk, sit in nature, practise yoga or meditate. It seems counterintuitive to 'slow down to speed up' – we get it!

The goal is to clear your mind of clutter so you can hear what's deep inside.

## Summary Points from Chapter 3 of *Ways to Quit Drinking*

- **Identify your 'why':** Understanding the underlying reasons for wanting to quit drinking is crucial. This chapter emphasises the importance of pinpointing your personal motivations to help you stay committed during challenging times.

- **Health and longevity:** Reflect on how alcohol consumption may be conflicting with your desire to live a long, healthy and active life. Consider the long-term health risks associated with drinking, including cancer, cognitive decline and poor sleep quality.

- **Quality of life:** Evaluate how alcohol affects your daily energy levels, productivity and overall wellbeing. Assess whether drinking is enhancing or detracting from your ability to live a vibrant, fulfilling life.

- **Positive role modelling:** Consider the impact of your drinking habits on those you influence, especially children and young people. Recognise the responsibility of setting a healthy example and how your behaviour can shape their future relationship with alcohol.

- **Nurturing relationships:** Examine how alcohol might be straining your close relationships, causing emotional distance and reducing the quality of your interactions with loved ones. Reflect on how quitting or reducing drinking could strengthen these connections.

- **Deep self-inquiry:** Engage in quiet, reflective practices to reconnect with your inner self and uncover the true motivators behind your desire to change your drinking habits. Use *self-inquiry* to reveal the subtleties of your needs and life path and support your continued growth and expansion.

In the words of spiritual mentor Akilesh Ayyar (2019, para. 39–40):

The idea of self-inquiry is that you are already what it is that you seek. The belief that you are a person, and all the desire-based thoughts, feelings, and actions based on that deeply-ingrained belief — those are the problem. They hide the fact of your true nature. They distract you from an underlying, constant peace.

So the question is how to get rid of those distractions. The answer is that you stop paying attention to them. And that happens over time. When you put in effort to inquire, you will eventually start to touch the real Self. It will be sweet enough that it will eventually become quite easy to stay there rather than allowing the mind to go chase so-called happiness elsewhere.

# Purpose of Workbook Chapter 3

When you are finished with Workbook Chapter 3, you will have:

- **Identified your core motivations:** You will have a clearer understanding of the fundamental reasons behind your desire to quit or reduce your drinking, recognising the personal significance of these motivations.

- **Assessed the health impacts:** You will have evaluated how alcohol consumption is affecting your health and longevity and understand the potential benefits of changing your drinking habits for a healthier future.

- **Reflected on your quality of life:** You will have considered the impact of alcohol on your daily energy levels, productivity and overall wellbeing, and how reducing or quitting can enhance your life's vibrancy.

- **Recognised your influence:** You will understand the importance of being a positive role model for those you influence and how your choices regarding alcohol can set a healthy example for others.

- **Examined your relationships:** You will have reflected on how alcohol may be affecting your close relationships and identified ways in which changing your drinking habits could strengthen these connections.

- **Clarified your 'why':** You will have developed a broad idea of your personal 'why' for exploring the option of quitting or reducing your drinking, with a commitment to refining and deepening this understanding if and as needed.

- **Planned for continued reflection:** You will be prepared to revisit and refine your motivations over time, recognising that this is an ongoing journey of self-discovery and growth.

# Exercises for Chapter 3

## *Exercise 1: Reflecting on Your Personal 'Why'*

1. **Quiet reflection time:** Find a quiet, comfortable space where you won't be interrupted. This could be a peaceful corner of your home, a favourite spot in nature or any place where you feel relaxed and at ease.

2. **Set the mood:** Create an atmosphere that encourages introspection. Light a candle, play calming music or use essential oils if they help you relax and focus.

3. **Journalling prompts:** Take out your journal or a piece of paper and write down the following questions:

    - Why am I considering reducing or quitting drinking?
    - What benefits do I hope to gain from making this change?
    - How does alcohol currently impact my health?
    - How does alcohol currently impact my relationships?
    - How does alcohol currently impact my overall quality of life?
    - What example do I want to set for others, especially those I care about?
    - What values and aspirations are important to me, and how does my relationship with alcohol align with these?

4. **Reflect and write:** Spend at least 20–30 minutes writing down your responses to these questions. Allow yourself to explore your thoughts and feelings honestly. Write freely without worrying about grammar or structure. Start with just single words, if that helps.

5. **Review and distil:** After you've finished writing, review your responses. Look for common themes, values and motivations that stand out to you. Circle or highlight key phrases or words that resonate deeply. Inexpensive coloured gel pens are fun for highlighting feelings, thoughts and inspiration.

6. **Identify your 'why':** Based on your reflections, distil your personal 'why' into a clear and definite statement that feels powerful to you. For example:

    - 'I want to demonstrate to my children that I can be fun and energetic and that a person doesn't have to drink to be the life of the party.'

    - 'I want to be walking the best of the world's famous hiking trails when I'm 70 and 80, so I need to be fit and healthy and free of chronic or life-threatening diseases.'

    - 'I am committed to being a role model for healthy living and inspiring those around me to live their best lives.'

    - 'I envisage a future where I'm fully present for my family, sharing meaningful moments without the distraction of alcohol.'

*Space for Reflection*

Why am I considering reducing or quitting drinking?

_____
_____
_____
_____
_____
_____
_____

What benefits do I hope to gain from making this change?

_____
_____
_____
_____
_____
_____
_____

How does alcohol currently impact my health?

_____
_____
_____
_____
_____
_____
_____

How does alcohol currently impact my relationships?

_____
_____
_____
_____
_____
_____
_____

How does alcohol currently impact my overall quality of life?

_____
_____
_____
_____
_____
_____
_____

What example do I want to set for others, especially those I care about?

_____
_____
_____
_____
_____
_____
_____

What values and aspirations are important to me, and how does my relationship with alcohol align with these?

_____
_____
_____
_____
_____
_____
_____

My 'why':

_____
_____
_____
_____
_____
_____
_____

## *Exercise 2: Visualisation and Future Pacing*

1. **Visualisation exercise:** Close your eyes and take several deep breaths to relax. Visualise yourself six months from now, having successfully reduced or quit drinking. Imagine your life and how it has improved as a result of this change.

2. **Imagine your ideal future:** Picture specific scenes in your mind:

    o **Health:** How do you feel physically and mentally?

    o **Relationships:** How have your relationships with loved ones improved?

    o **Daily life:** What activities are you now able to enjoy more fully?

    o **Personal growth:** How have you grown as a person?

3. **Journal your vision (write down your vision in words):** Open your eyes and write down a detailed description of the future you envisage:

    o Describe how your life has changed for the better since reducing or quitting drinking.

    o Reflect on the specific benefits you are experiencing in terms of health, relationships and personal fulfilment.

4. **Identify your motivation:** After visualising and journalling, identify the key motivations that have emerged from this exercise. What values and aspirations are driving your desire to make this change?

5. **Commitment statement:** Write a commitment statement based on your vision and motivations. For example:

    - 'I am committed to consuming only healthy foods and beverages to optimise my health and live the longest and most vibrant life I can.'

    - 'I am committed to working on healthy ways to deal with my thoughts and emotions rather than self-medicating with alcohol.'

    - 'I am committed to quitting drinking to be present for my children and strengthen my relationship with them.'

6. **Review and refine:** Review your commitment statement and make any necessary adjustments. Keep it somewhere visible as a reminder of your 'why' and your commitment to making positive changes in your life.

*Space for Reflection*

**Imagine your ideal future:** Picture the following specific scenes in your mind:

*(**Tip:** Write as though you are there, now, experiencing that future moment.)*

**Health:** How do you feel physically and mentally?

_____
_____
_____
_____
_____
_____
_____

**Relationships:** How have your relationships with loved ones improved?

_____
_____
_____
_____
_____

**Daily life:** What activities are you now able to enjoy more fully?

_____
_____
_____
_____
_____
_____
_____

**Personal growth:** How have you grown as a person?

_____
_____
_____
_____
_____
_____
_____

**Journal your vision:** Open your eyes and write down a detailed description of the future you envisage:

*(**Tip:** Write as though you are there, now, experiencing that future moment.)*

Describe how your life has changed for the better since reducing or quitting drinking.

_____
_____
_____
_____
_____
_____
_____

Reflect on the specific benefits you are experiencing in terms of health, relationships and personal fulfilment.

___

**Identify your motivation:** What values and aspirations are driving your desire to make this change?

___

**Commitment statement:** Write a commitment statement based on your vision and motivations.

___

## *Summary of the Two Exercises*

While both exercises aim to help you discover your 'why' for changing your drinking habits, Exercise 1 is more about introspection and self-reflection while Exercise 2 uses visualisation and future imagining to reinforce your motivations with positive imagery and experiences. Exercise 2 builds upon Exercise 1 but approaches discovering your 'why' from a different angle. Here's how they differ:

- **Exercise 1 (Reflecting on Your Personal 'Why'):**
    - In Exercise 1, you engage in quiet reflection and journalling to explore your motivations for wanting to quit or reduce drinking.
    - It focuses on asking specific questions and prompting you to write about your thoughts and feelings related to your relationship with alcohol.
    - The goal is to distil your personal 'why' into a clear statement that resonates with you.

- **Exercise 2 (Visualisation and Future Pacing):**
    - Exercise 2 involves visualisation and future pacing to imagine yourself six months from now, having successfully reduced or quit drinking.
    - You visualise specific scenes in your ideal future, focusing on how your life has improved as a result of making this change.
    - It asks you to journal about the future you envisage and reflect on the benefits you are experiencing in terms of health, relationships and personal growth.
    - The goal is to solidify your commitment and motivation by visualising the positive outcomes of changing your relationship with alcohol.

They complement each other by offering different perspectives and methods to explore your motivations.

## Notes

# Chapter 4:

# Breaking Free From Alcohol – A Practical Look at Ways to Stop Drinking – Applying It to Your Life

## Overview

Chapter 4 explores the theme of 'Breaking Free From Alcohol – A Practical Look at Ways to Stop Drinking'. This chapter presents what can be a transformative journey for the millions of people worldwide who are seeking to overcome alcohol dependence. It challenges individuals to confront not only their reliance on alcohol but also the emotional, social and psychological factors that contribute to it.

Throughout this chapter, we delve into a diverse range of approaches to quitting drinking, examining the potential benefits and drawbacks of each. From the long-standing tradition of Alcoholics Anonymous (AA) to the 'cold turkey' method, medication-assisted treatments, nutritional therapies and holistic lifestyle changes, each approach offers unique perspectives, strategies and support systems. We will explore the fundamental beliefs, processes and practices that underpin each method, backed by scientific evidence and real-world implications.

By studying Chapter 4 of *Ways to Quit Drinking*, you will gain insights into these approaches and a closer understanding of their effectiveness and limitations. This exploration will empower you with the knowledge to make better-informed decisions about some of the options available to you on your path to a healthier future, free from a dependence on alcohol.

# Reading Assignment, Chapter 4

Read Chapter 4 of Ways to Quit Drinking: A Sober Curious Book on How to Control Alcohol for Better Health, Self-Esteem and Mental Clarity.

Note: You will no doubt notice that our list of strategies for quitting drinking does not include options like inpatient and outpatient treatment programmes and other not-for-profit and community-based programmes. There are two reasons for this. One reason is that we do not have first-hand experience of attending these types of programmes as either they were not available or we did not know of them, or did not know how to get sufficiently detailed information about them. The second reason is that it's not realistically possible to cover all available options. The strategies we've covered here serve to highlight the critical elements you should seek out to be sure you cover all the needs you will have on your journey. It's a place to start, you might say!

## Summary Points From Chapter 4 of *Ways to Quit Drinking*

1. **Alcoholics Anonymous (AA)**
    - **Description:** AA is a globally renowned mutual aid fellowship founded in 1935, offering support and guidance to individuals struggling with alcohol addiction through a 12-step programme. It emphasises mutual support, admitting powerlessness over alcohol, surrendering to a higher power and taking personal inventory.
    - **Core philosophy:** Abstinence from alcohol as the foundation for recovery, anonymity, mutual support and sponsorship.
    - **Structure:** Decentralised, with over 115,000 autonomous groups worldwide, meeting in various settings.
    - **Key features:** Sponsorship system, regular meetings and AA literature (*Big Book* and *Twelve Steps and Twelve Traditions*).

    **Pros:**
    - **Peer support:** Offers a judgement-free community for individuals facing alcohol dependence, fostering camaraderie and social motivation.

- Twelve-step programme: Structured pathway to sobriety through self-reflection, surrender and restitution, guided by sponsors.

- Anonymity: Promotes honest sharing and accountability within a confidential setting.

- Sponsorship: Personal mentorship from experienced members helps newcomers navigate challenges.

- Spiritual growth: Encourages seeking support from a higher power, promoting personal growth beyond alcohol.

- Regular meetings: Provides consistent community support and encouragement.

- Personal accountability: Emphasises taking responsibility for past errors and making amends.

- Long-term sobriety success stories: Inspires hope and resilience through real-life examples.

- Inclusive atmosphere: Welcomes people from diverse backgrounds in a supportive environment.

- Accessibility: Offers global and virtual meetings for consistent support.

**Cons:**

- Spiritual emphasis: Focus on a higher power may conflict with non-traditional beliefs.

- Focus on powerlessness: Emphasis on surrender may deter those seeking empowerment and autonomy.

- One-size-fits-all approach: Lack of flexibility in the structured programme may not suit individuals with complex needs.

- Lack of professional therapy: Relies on peer support rather than professional clinical treatment.

- Anonymity challenges: Risk of breaches in closely connected communities, deterring some individuals from participation.

- Reliance on meetings: Requires regular attendance, which can be challenging for those with transportation or schedule barriers.

- **No formal research basis:** Lack of scientific research on effectiveness compared to other treatment methods.

- **Criticisms of effectiveness:** Long-term success rates are lower than for other evidence-based treatments, raising questions about overall effectiveness.

Overall, while AA provides a supportive community and a methodical approach to recovery, its structured programme and emphasis on spiritual surrender may not align with everyone's needs,. Some individuals may benefit from a combination of AA and professional therapy for more comprehensive support.

2. **Cold turkey**

    - **Description:** Cold turkey involves the abrupt and complete cessation of alcohol consumption without a gradual reduction or any professional intervention.

    - **Approach:** Self-directed, often the result of a sudden decision to stop drinking.

**Pros:**

- **Immediate action and increased motivation:** Makes a decisive commitment to an alcohol-free life, empowering and motivating rapid change.

- **Clear break:** Provides a distinct mental and emotional break from alcohol dependence.

- **Rapid detoxification:** Allows for quicker elimination of alcohol from the body, potentially reducing withdrawal symptoms sooner.

- **Potential for quick results:** Can lead to rapid improvements in physical health, mental clarity and overall wellbeing.

- **Self-directed independence:** Empowers individuals to take personal responsibility and make independent health choices.

- **Cost-effective:** Does not involve the expense of formal treatment programmes or rehabilitation centres.

- **Avoidance of gradual reduction challenges:** Simplifies the process by eliminating the need for complex tapering schedules.

- **Personal transformation:** Acts as a catalyst for profound lifestyle changes and positive habits.

**Cons:**

- **Potential for intense withdrawal symptoms and health risks:** May lead to severe withdrawal symptoms like anxiety, insomnia, tremors and even seizures, with the latter requiring medical attention.

- **Increased risk of relapse:** Higher likelihood of relapse due to severe withdrawal symptoms and persistent cravings, especially in the first few weeks.

- **Managing psychological challenges:** Can trigger mood swings, irritability, anxiety, depression and stress without professional support.

- **Lack of professional guidance:** Lacks the structured guidance and coping strategies provided by professional treatment programmes.

- **Doesn't consider the whole person:** Fails to address nutritional deficiencies and the overall health restoration necessary for sustained abstinence.

- **Research basis:** While effective in the long run for some, this approach lacks formal scientific research on its overall effectiveness compared to other methods.

Overall, quitting cold turkey can be empowering and may lead to quick improvements, but it also carries significant risks and challenges, particularly for heavy drinkers. Seeking professional advice and care is crucial, especially for those with severe alcohol dependence.

3. **Willpower**

    - **Description:** Willpower refers to the mental strength and determination to resist the urge to drink alcohol and maintain an alcohol-free life.

    - **Approach:** Self-control, making a firm decision to change behaviour.

    - **Strategies:** Exercising self-control, resisting triggers, staying goal-oriented and building mental strength.

**Pros:**

- **Independence and flexibility:** Allows for a personal plan and timeline for quitting without the need for external programmes or apps.

- **Intrinsic motivation and ownership:** Taps into inner motivations, making the decision to quit feel like a personal choice, thereby enhancing dedication.

- **Self-discipline and responsibility:** Builds self-control and accountability, promoting personal development and healthier decision-making.

- **Personal development:** Promotes growth, resilience and self-reflection, fostering coping mechanisms and the exploration of healthier lifestyles.

- **Long-term empowerment:** Boosts confidence and belief in oneself, providing ongoing empowerment and personal growth.

**Cons:**

- **Limited resource:** Willpower is finite and can be depleted, leading to mental fatigue and reduced ability to cope with stress or triggers.

- **Unlikely to address root causes:** Does not resolve underlying emotional or mental issues that most likely contribute to problem drinking.

- **Limited coping mechanisms:** Without strategies to manage stress and triggers, reliance on willpower alone can be mentally exhausting.

- **Vulnerability to triggers and relapse:** High-stress situations can challenge willpower, increasing the risk of relapse without adequate coping strategies.

- **Potential for negative self-image:** Reliance on willpower alone may lead to self-blame and setbacks, hindering progress and perpetuating the cycle of drinking.

- **Overemphasis on individual effort:** Ignores the benefits of external assistance, such as peer support and guidance, which can be crucial for long-term abstinence.

While willpower is valuable for abstaining from alcohol, its limitations mean that a multifaceted approach addressing physical, mental and emotional aspects is often more successful. For severe alcohol dependence, medical intervention and comprehensive treatment programmes may be necessary in addition to willpower.

4. **Vitamin therapy**

    - **Description:** Using nutritional supplements, such as vitamins and minerals, to address deficiencies caused by chronic alcohol use and support recovery.

    - **Approach:** Orthomolecular medicine, replenishing nutrients to counteract cravings and withdrawal effects.

    - **Evidence:** Research suggests potential benefits in reducing cravings and supporting recovery.

**Pros:**

- **Nutrient support:** Provides essential vitamins and minerals to replenish deficiencies caused by heavy alcohol consumption, supporting overall health and wellbeing.

- **Brain health:** Certain vitamins, especially B vitamins, aid in brain function and mood regulation, potentially assisting in neurological recovery post-alcohol dependence.

- **Reduced cravings:** Vitamin B3 (niacin) has been noted to help alleviate alcohol cravings during early abstinence, potentially aiding in the transition to sobriety.

- **Cellular repair:** Antioxidants in vitamins help repair the cell damage caused by alcohol toxins, potentially reducing discomfort and fatigue during recovery.

- **Relief of withdrawal symptoms:** Comprehensive nutritional support may stabilise mood, digestion, sleep and cognition, while specific supplements can address withdrawal symptoms like anxiety and muscle tension.

**Cons:**

- **Lack of scientific consensus:** Vitamin therapy lacks large-scale studies proving its effectiveness and remains controversial in mainstream medicine despite personal anecdotes of benefit.

- o **Individual variability:** Vitamin needs and responses vary widely among individuals, requiring personalised approaches that may not work universally.

- o **Potential safety issues:** Some would say that megadosing vitamins can pose risks, particularly if self-prescribed without medical guidance. Interactions with medications or health conditions need consideration.

- o **Delaying comprehensive care:** While nutrition supports overall wellness, relying solely on vitamin therapy may delay the holistic care needed for long-term sobriety.

- o **Financial commitment:** Professional-grade supplements are costly and often not covered by insurance, limiting accessibility for those with financial constraints.

- o **Risks of self-treatment:** Self-prescribing vitamin regimens based on internet research without medical oversight can be risky, potentially leading to adverse effects.

In summary, while vitamin therapy offers potential benefits for addressing nutrient deficiencies and supporting recovery from alcohol dependence, it should be approached cautiously due to the lack of robust scientific evidence and the need for personalised, medically supervised treatment plans. Always consult with healthcare professionals before adopting any new treatment approach.

5. **Medication-assisted treatment (MAT)**

- o **Description:** Evidence-based treatment combining medications (e.g., disulfiram, naltrexone, acamprosate) with counselling and therapy to manage cravings and support recovery.

- o **Approach:** Individualised treatment plans based on addiction severity and co-occurring disorders.

**Pros:**

- o **Research-backed effectiveness:** Extensive studies demonstrate that MAT, when combined with counselling and behavioural therapies, improves treatment outcomes and long-term recovery rates.

- o **Reduced cravings and withdrawal symptoms:** Medications like naltrexone and acamprosate help reduce alcohol cravings, alleviate withdrawal symptoms and block the pleasurable effects of alcohol.

- **Improved treatment adherence and outcomes:** MAT enhances treatment adherence, reduces the risk of relapse and can be part of a long-term strategy for maintaining recovery.

- **Integrated approach:** By combining medication with counselling and therapy, MAT comprehensively addresses both the physical and psychological aspects of addiction.

- **Individualised treatment:** MAT allows for tailored treatment plans based on each individual's needs, optimising treatment effectiveness.

- **Improved quality of life:** MAT has been shown to increase engagement with treatment, reduce alcohol-related problems and enhance quality of life compared to treatments without medication.

**Cons:**

- **Potential side effects:** Medications used in MAT can cause side effects ranging from mild to severe, depending on the medication and individual response.

- **Stigma and hesitance:** Some individuals may be hesitant to use medications due to stigma or a preference for abstinence-only approaches.

- **Adherence risk:** There is a risk of non-adherence to the medication regimen, which can reduce its effectiveness.

- **Cost and accessibility limitations:** MAT may be limited by cost and accessibility issues, depending on insurance coverage and treatment setting.

- **Potential drug interactions:** Medications used in MAT can interact with other drugs, necessitating careful management by healthcare providers.

- **Variable effectiveness:** MAT may not work for everyone with alcohol use disorder (AUD), as treatment outcomes can vary based on individual factors.

- **Potential for over-reliance:** There is a risk of relying too heavily on medication and not addressing the underlying behavioural, psychological and social aspects of addiction through counselling and therapy.

- **Risk of continued drinking:** MAT can reduce cravings and support abstinence, but it does not guarantee that individuals won't drink.

In summary, MAT is an evidence-based treatment approach that combines medications with counselling and therapy to effectively address alcohol addiction. While it offers significant benefits, such as reduced cravings and improved treatment adherence, it also comes with considerations like potential side effects, adherence issues and the need for comprehensive treatment planning. Open communication with healthcare providers is crucial to determine if MAT is an appropriate choice and to optimise its effectiveness.

6. **Guidance through coaching, counselling or therapy**

    - **Description:** Professional support from coaches, counsellors or therapists to provide guidance, coping strategies and accountability.
    - **Approach:** Collaborative and goal-oriented, addressing underlying issues and developing skills for managing stress and cravings.
    - **Professionals:** Psychologists, social workers, licensed professional counsellors (LPCs), marriage and family therapists (MFTs) and addiction specialists.

**Pros:**

- **Personalised support:** Offers tailored assistance based on individual circumstances, needs and goals, ensuring relevant and targeted support.
- **Moral support:** Provides emotional encouragement and understanding, fostering a sense of companionship and motivation throughout the journey.
- **Accountability:** Regular check-ins and goal setting ensure commitment and progress, enhancing motivation and adherence.
- **Insights into emotional wellbeing:** Provides a safe space for self-reflection, gaining insights into triggers, patterns and emotional issues contributing to drinking.
- **Coping strategies and guidance:** Promotes techniques for managing stress, anxiety and triggers without alcohol, developing essential skills for long-term resilience.
- **Neuroplasticity and brain rewiring:** Therapeutic techniques promote healthier habits and emotional regulation through neural pathway rewiring.

- **Goal achievement:** Setting and working towards specific, achievable goals related to maintaining an alcohol-free lifestyle.
- **Holistic approach:** Addresses physical, emotional and psychological aspects for comprehensive recovery and wellbeing.
- **Confidentiality:** Private, secure environment for open and honest conversations without fear of judgement.
- **Professional expertise:** Provides access to specialised knowledge and experience in addiction, recovery and mental health from trained professionals.
- **Long-term success:** Builds a foundation for sustained abstinence and overall wellbeing through personal growth and coping strategies.

**Cons:**

- **Medical record implications:** Potential documentation of mental health or addiction issues, raising concerns about future implications.
- **High expenses:** Costly sessions, potentially limiting access to this type of support or causing financial stress.
- **Variation in approach:** Different professionals may have varying effectiveness and approaches, requiring trial and error to find the best fit.
- **Limited personal understanding:** Lack of personal experience or deep empathy from professionals, potentially affecting relatability and outcomes.
- **Admitting to a stranger:** Emotional barriers may hinder openness and progress due to feelings of humiliation or shame.
- **Communication barriers:** Challenges in expressing thoughts and feelings verbally, potentially impacting session effectiveness.
- **Limited availability:** Scheduling constraints and availability issues due to cost or practitioner availability, delaying needed support.
- **Compatibility issues:** Effectiveness depends on the match between the individual and the professional, impacting trust and comfort in the therapeutic relationship.

- o **Lack of peer support:** Absence of the communal understanding and peer support found in group settings, potentially limiting effectiveness.

- o **Limited perspective:** Reliance on one professional's perspective may overlook alternative approaches that could be beneficial.

In summary, seeking guidance through coaching, counselling or therapy provides personalised support, accountability and coping strategies crucial for quitting drinking. However, potential drawbacks like cost, varied effectiveness and personal barriers should be considered when choosing this approach. It's essential to find a supportive professional and be aware of the potential challenges to maximise the benefits of this option.

7. **Self-help books and resources**

   - o **Description:** Resources beyond professional help, including self-help books, online courses and community support groups.

   - o **Approach:** Educational platforms and virtual communities providing insights, advice and moral support.

   - o **Accessibility:** Widely available and accessible resources for those seeking an alcohol-free lifestyle.

**Pros:**

- o **Abundance of published books:** Thousands of self-help books offer diverse perspectives, strategies and personal narratives, available in various formats (physical, ebooks, audiobooks) and accessible at affordable prices.

- o **Diversity in approaches and accessibility:** Wide range of resources, including books, blogs, online courses, apps, hotlines and community support groups, catering to different preferences and needs.

- o **Global reach and community engagement:** Online sobriety communities on platforms like Facebook connect individuals globally, offering support groups tailored by gender, age and method, fostering a sense of community and understanding.

- o **Broadening visibility, embracing 'sober curious':** Increased visibility and acceptance of sobriety and the alcohol-free lifestyle, including the 'sober curious' movement, promoting alternative paths to sobriety and enriching recovery discourse.

- **Global participation in alcohol-free challenges:** International events like 'Dry January' and 'Sober October' encourage collective periods of alcohol abstinence, fostering global camaraderie and shared goals.
- **Rise of alcohol-free drinks:** Growing market for alcohol-free options, reflecting increased health consciousness and providing social alternatives without the negative effects of alcohol.

Cons:

- **Varied quality and intent of resources:** Quality and biases vary among resources, requiring careful selection; some may push additional products or services.
- **Potential lack of professional guidance:** Lack of direct oversight and personalised guidance from professionals like coaches or therapists may mean complex individual needs are not addressed.
- **Isolation and limited peer support:** Relying solely on self-help methods may lead to feelings of isolation due to the absence of peer support found in group settings.
- **Risk for individuals with high dependency:** For those with severe alcohol dependency, relying solely on self-help methods without medical supervision can be risky, especially regarding withdrawal symptoms and medical complications.

In summary, self-help books and resources provide a wide range of accessible options and community support for individuals seeking to quit drinking, but potential drawbacks include varying quality, lack of professional guidance, isolation and risks for those with high dependency. It's important to approach these resources with discernment and consider additional support from healthcare professionals when needed.

8. **A holistic approach to lifestyle transformation**

    - **Description:** Comprehensive approach addressing genetic, neurobiological, emotional coping, habitual and environmental factors influencing alcohol dependence.
    - **Approach:** Focuses on lifestyle changes, mindfulness and personal growth practices.
    - **Components:** Nutrition, physical activity, sleep hygiene, emotional wellbeing (mindfulness, emotional freedom technique [EFT] tapping,

congitive behavioural therapy [CBT]), engaging hobbies and tracking progress.

**Pros:**

- **Addresses root causes:** Tackles genetic, neurobiological, emotional and habitual factors, offering a comprehensive and sustainable solution.

- **Empowers the individual:** Equips people with tools to manage their alcohol-free journey independently.

- **Enhances overall health and wellbeing:** Focuses on optimal physical health through nutrition, exercise and sleep.

- **Develops emotional resilience:** Integrates practices like mindfulness, EFT and CBT to manage stress and negative emotions.

- **Fosters personal growth:** Promotes self-awareness, healthier habits and improvements in self-esteem and relationships.

- **Flexible and customisable:** Tailored to individual needs, preferences and circumstances.

- **Provides long-term benefits:** Offers sustainable benefits by addressing underlying issues and developing healthy coping mechanisms.

- **Encourages self-reflection and mindfulness:** Promotes self-awareness and mindfulness, aiding in maintaining good mental health.

- **A proactive approach:** Focuses on prevention and wellness, empowering individuals to take charge of their health.

**Cons:**

- **Requires commitment and effort:** Changing habits and maintaining motivation can be challenging.

- **May be time-consuming:** Implementing lifestyle changes and engaging in new activities can require significant time and energy.

- **Can be emotionally challenging:** Confronting emotional issues and learning new coping strategies can be taxing.

- **Requires patience and persistence:** Results may be gradual, requiring perseverance to see full benefits.

- o **May require professional support:** Severe cases may need additional professional help, which can be costly and time-consuming.

- o **Risk of relapse:** Despite efforts to reduce risk, the possibility of relapse exists, requiring ongoing vigilance and support.

- o **Potential for overwhelming changes:** Overhauling multiple aspects of life simultaneously can feel overwhelming.

- o **Requires self-motivation:** Personal accountability is essential, which can be challenging for some.

- o **May not be sufficient for severe cases:** For severe alcohol dependence, additional medical intervention may be necessary.

This summary encapsulates the main points from the holistic approach to quitting drinking, highlighting both the benefits and potential challenges.

# Purpose of Workbook Chapter 4

After reading Chapter 4, here are the main takeaways you will have:

- **Wider understanding of the options:** You will likely have gained a comprehensive understanding of the various approaches available for quitting drinking, ranging from traditional methods like AA to newer approaches like vitamin therapy and holistic lifestyle changes.

- **Personalisation of approach:** You will be sure to recognise the importance of choosing an approach that aligns with your individual needs, preferences and circumstances.

- **Empowerment through knowledge:** You will likely feel more empowered by having knowledge of the different strategies and tools that can support your journey towards an alcohol-free lifestyle.

- **Holistic approach:** You will appreciate the value of a holistic approach that considers multiple factors influencing alcohol dependence, including genetics, neurobiology, emotional coping mechanisms, habits and environmental influences.

- **Hope and possibility:** The chapter will instil a sense of hope and possibility by demonstrating that there are effective methods and resources available to help you overcome an unhealthy relationship with alcohol.

- **Practical steps:** You will find practical steps and actionable advice on how to implement each approach, whether it's seeking professional help, joining a support group or making lifestyle changes.

- **Importance of support:** You will understand the importance of support networks, whether through professional counsellors, support groups or personal coaches, in maintaining motivation and accountability.

- **Long-term recovery:** You will appreciate the goal of long-term recovery and how each approach contributes to building a stable and alcohol-free life.

- **Mindset shift:** You will ideally have undergone a mindset shift, from feeling overwhelmed by a problematic relationship with alcohol to feeling hopeful and proactive about your future.

- **Inspiration for action:** Finally, we hope you will be inspired to take action, knowing that there are multiple pathways to quitting drinking and achieving a healthier, more fulfilling life.

These takeaways aim to provide you with a clear understanding of your options and inspire you to choose a path that best suits your needs, setting the stage for successful extrication from alcohol dependence and a move towards personal growth.

# Exercise for Chapter 4

## *Exercise 1: Which Option Will You Adopt?*

Based on the options detailed in this book, as well as any other options you may know about – such as local community groups, online informal chat and support groups and proprietary methods (e.g., The Sinclair Method, SMART Recovery) – what are the options open to you?

Take into account your schedule and time availability (e.g., do you have time in the evenings to go to meetings?), your budget (e.g., can you pay for a coach or treatment programme?) and the availability of moral and emotional support and your degree of need for it (i.e., does no one else around you drink and they'll support you to give up, *or* does everyone else around you drink and you'll need some strong and present support to keep you strong?).

Write down what your intention is regarding your options for quitting:

_____
_____
_____
_____
_____
_____
_____
_____
_____
_____
_____
_____
_____
_____
_____
_____
_____

## Notes

_____
_____
_____
_____
_____
_____
_____
_____
_____

# Chapter 5:

# When You Know You Need to Stop Drinking – Applying It to Your Life

## Overview

In this chapter, we enter a pivotal phase of your journey towards an alcohol-free life: the realisation that it's time to make a change. Recognising that drinking has become problematic is a courageous and essential step. We explore the personal and societal influences that often keep us stuck in unhealthy patterns and how reaching a turning point can shift your perspective. By sharing personal experiences and guiding you through a series of reflective questions, this chapter helps you confront the reality of your relationship with alcohol and envisage a healthier future.

This chapter is structured around three critical steps that guide you through this process.

### *Step 1: Realisation That There Is a Problem*

Understanding the impact of alcohol on your life requires deep introspection and honesty. This step provides a framework to evaluate your drinking habits, the consequences you've faced and how alcohol aligns with your values and goals. By answering reflective questions, you'll gain valuable insights into your relationship with alcohol and any patterns around its use.

### *Step 2: Information Gathering, Decision Time and Action Time*

Armed with the insights from Step 1, you'll gather additional information and reflect on the knowledge shared in previous chapters. This step is about making an informed decision: whether to cut back, abstain for a set period or quit entirely. You'll weigh the pros and cons, consider your past attempts at moderation and decide the best path forward.

## Step 3: Managing the Decision Long-Term

Making the decision to change is only the beginning. In this step, you'll explore practical strategies for maintaining your decision, including handling cravings, navigating social situations and building a supportive environment. This step is about preparing for the challenges ahead and ensuring your commitment to a healthier, alcohol-free life.

By the end of this chapter, you'll be better equipped to make a clear, informed decision about your relationship with alcohol and take actionable steps towards a transformative and fulfilling alcohol-free life.

# Reading Assignment, Chapter 5

Read Chapter 5 of Ways to Quit Drinking: A Sober Curious Book on How to Control Alcohol for Better Health, Self-Esteem and Mental Clarity.

There is a lot of information in this chapter! Much of it is very exciting (if you choose to approach it that way...) because it provides an opportunity to contemplate a myriad of ways to move forward, well-armed with answers, options and ideas.

Quitting drinking isn't just a matter of 'last drink' and then nothing. That simply leaves a person 'high and dry' with no support or coping mechanisms. This chapter helps you explore and choose elements to create your healthier future, filled with more certainty and tools to guard against setbacks. Approach this chapter with an open mind and consider all the possibilities.

# Summary Points from Chapter 5 of *Ways to Quit Drinking*

- **Realisation of the problem:** Understanding that moderation isn't working and recognising that the pervasive influence of cultural and societal conditioning on your drinking habits – which are possibly overlaying genetic and personality-based factors, among others – means alcohol is robbing you of your best life.

- **Personal turning point:** Identifying the moment when – or gradual dawning of the realisation that – the pain of drinking outweighs the fear of missing out, leading to the decision to make a change in your relationship with alcohol.

- **Critical questions to contemplate:** Reflecting on personal drinking patterns, consequences, struggles with moderation and the impact of alcohol on physical and mental wellbeing, relationships and long-term goals.

- **Decision time:** Considering three main options for moving forward – cutting back, abstaining for good or abstaining for a set period – based on personal reflections and past experiences with moderation. *Where do you want to be 12 months from now?*

- **Action plan:** Preparing to implement your decision by developing a clear plan, identifying a support system and addressing potential challenges such as handling cravings, social situations and managing relationships with people who still drink.

# Purpose of Workbook Chapter 5

After reading Workbook Chapter 5, you will have the know-how to:

- **Recognise the signs:** You will understand how to identify the signs that indicate your drinking is problematic and why recognising these signs is a crucial first step towards change.

- **Reflect on personal experiences:** You will have gained insights into your own drinking habits and patterns, including difficulties with moderation and the impact on various aspects of your life.

- **Ask critical questions:** You will have taken the time to contemplate and honestly answer critical questions about your drinking, including the effects on your physical and mental health, relationships and long-term goals.

- **Explore options for change:** You will have assessed the different potential paths forward – cutting back, abstaining permanently or abstaining temporarily – and understand the importance of choosing the right option for your unique situation.

- **Prepare for action:** You will have developed a concrete action plan for moving forward, including setting clear goals, identifying support systems and planning for potential challenges and setbacks.

- **Build confidence in your decision-making:** You will feel empowered and confident in your ability to make informed decisions about your relationship with alcohol and understand that you have the strength and resources to create a healthier, alcohol-free future.

# Exercises for Chapter 5

## *Step 1: Realisation That There Is a Problem*

*Exercise 1: Answer these critical questions:*

1. How often do you find yourself exceeding your intended limit when drinking?

_____
_____
_____
_____

Consider this carefully. If you set out to have just one glass, how many more than this intended amount would you normally have? Be honest with yourself about your patterns.

_____
_____
_____
_____

2. Have you faced negative personal or professional consequences because of your drinking?

_____
_____
_____
_____

Have you called in sick to work because you were hungover?

_____
_____
_____
_____

Have you missed important conference sessions, events or appointments after overindulging the night before?

_____
_____
_____
_____

Have you felt unwell while getting the kids to school after drinking too much? Or 'suffered' while carrying out normal daily responsibilities?

_____
_____
_____
_____

These are all red flags.

3. When trying to cut back, do you struggle to consistently stick to your limits?

_____
_____
_____
_____

Government health departments recommend having a few alcohol-free days per week. You can check out the guidelines from health departments around the world here:

- **National Institute on Alcohol Abuse and Alcoholism (USA):** www.niaaa.nih.gov/alcohol-health/overview-alcohol-consumption/moderate-binge-drinking

- **Drinkaware (UK):** www.drinkaware.co.uk/facts/information-about-alcohol/alcohol-and-the-facts/low-risk-drinking-guidelines

- **Canadian Centre on Substance Abuse and Addiction:** www.ccsa.ca/canadas-guidance-alcohol-and-health

- **National Health and Medical Research Council (Australia):** www.nhmrc.gov.au/health-advice/alcohol

Can you stick within these limits? Or do you find yourself drinking daily because abstaining is too hard?

_____
_____
_____
_____

*A share: We found we couldn't stick to these recommendations. In fact, I'd go so far as to say that if we had limited ourselves to these recommendations, we would have considered that 'barely a drink' and that it probably didn't count!*

Just as it was for us, an inability to stick within these guidelines is a sign that your drinking is becoming a dependency.

4. How does alcohol impact your physical and mental wellbeing?

_____
_____
_____

Do you often feel sick, unwell or hungover after drinking?

_____
_____
_____
_____

Do you worry about your alcohol intake? (Do you often ask yourself questions like 'Am I drinking more than others?', 'Does anyone else drink as much as I do?' or 'How will I know if I'm doing myself damage?')

_____
_____
_____
_____

Do you notice that emotional issues seem to worsen over time when you're drinking regularly?

_____
_____
_____
_____

5. Have loved ones expressed concern about your drinking habits? Sometimes those closest to us notice things before we're ready to admit them to ourselves.

_____
_____
_____
_____

Have you noticed your partner, family or friends glancing at your glass as you pour another drink, even if they don't say anything? They may be worried about you.

_____
_____
_____
_____

6. Have you noticed increased tolerance – needing more alcohol for the same effects?

___

Tolerance is a clear sign that your body is adapting to alcohol.

Think about times when you've had a period of abstinence. Do you initially feel satisfied with less alcohol, but within a month or two find yourself wanting to drink more to get the same 'buzz'?

___

7. How does your alcohol use align with your personal values and long-term goals?

___

Think carefully about this, and about the facts we've covered so far:

- Chapter 1 detailed alcohol's capabilities and uses

- Chapter 2 explained why people develop drinking problems
- Chapter 3 looked at reasons for considering quitting

Now, consider your own drinking habits.

Does your current alcohol use truly align with your values and goals? Or are you experiencing cognitive dissonance – the mental discomfort that arises when your beliefs and behaviours are in conflict?

_____
_____
_____
_____
_____
_____
_____
_____
_____

8. Have you tried moderating your drinking before and, if so, what were the results?

_____
_____
_____
_____
_____
_____
_____
_____
_____

Many people try to cut back on their drinking before they consider quitting entirely.

If you've tried this, how did it go?

Were you able to easily have drink-free days each week?

Could you take or leave alcohol without worry?

Or did you feel agitated and go to great lengths to get the alcohol you wanted?

Be honest about your past attempts.

_____
_____
_____
_____
_____
_____
_____
_____
_____

9. How do you feel about the idea of abstaining from alcohol for a set period, like one month?

_____
_____
_____
_____
_____
_____
_____
_____
_____

Challenges like 'Dry January' or 'Sober October' have become popular in recent years. Have you ever attempted one of these?

_____
_____
_____
_____

How does the thought of taking on such a challenge make you feel? Excited and motivated? Or filled with apprehension and dread?

_____
_____
_____
_____
_____
_____
_____
_____

Your reaction can tell you a lot.

Research a few of these initiatives – you may find inspiration and support in the community surrounding the events. Here's some to get you started:

- **Dry January:** A month-long challenge in January to abstain from alcohol, initiated by Alcohol Change UK. https://alcoholchange.org.uk/help-and-support/managing-your-drinking/dry-january

- **FebFast:** A challenge in February to give up alcohol (and sometimes sugar or other vices) to raise funds for youth addiction services. https://febfast.org.au/

- **Dry July:** A challenge to abstain from alcohol during July to raise funds for cancer patients. https://www.dryjuly.com/

- **Sober October:** A challenge to stay sober during October, often linked to fundraising for various charities. https://www.gosober.org.uk/

- **Sober Spring:** A challenge to abstain from alcohol for the entire spring season, providing a longer-term commitment to sobriety. https://alcoholchange.org.uk/help-and-support/managing-your-drinking/sober-spring

There are others, but you get the idea! Gearing up for a 21-day reset or a 30-day challenge, or even a 100-day no alcohol commitment, can be a goal you set yourself at any time. Even better – if you know others who would like to do a 'detox' to clean up their act, you could embark on something like this together!

_____
_____
_____
_____
_____
_____
_____
_____
_____
_____
_____
_____

10. Can you envisage a positive, fulfilling life without relying on alcohol?

_____
_____
_____
_____
_____
_____
_____
_____

Are you a prime example of being a product of your environmental conditioning and the alcohol-centric culture you are immersed in?

What do you perceive you will miss out on as a non-drinker?

_____
_____
_____
_____
_____
_____
_____
_____
_____

*Exercise 2: Pros vs. Cons*

Do the cons of drinking outweigh the pros when you think about your long-term goals and values?

List what you think the benefits of quitting drinking will be for you, and also list the downsides you believe you will experience as a non-drinker.

| Benefits of becoming a non-drinker | Downsides of becoming a non-drinker |
|---|---|
|  |  |
|  |  |
|  |  |
|  |  |
|  |  |
|  |  |
|  |  |
|  |  |
|  |  |
|  |  |
|  |  |
|  |  |

## Step 2: Information Gathering, Decision Time and Action Time

### Exercise 3: Decision

Circle the option you plan to adopt:

| Choice 1: | Choice 2: | Choice 3: |
|---|---|---|
| Choose to cut back | Choose to abstain for good | Choose to abstain for a set period of time |

## Step 3: Managing the Decision Long-Term

### Exercise 4: Filling Your Toolbox

See Step 3 in Chapter 5 of *Ways to Quit Drinking* for lists of ideas to choose from.

This is what I plan to drink instead:

_____
_____
_____
_____
_____
_____

This is what I plan to do at 'that time of day':

_____
_____
_____
_____
_____
_____

This is what I will do at social occasions when everyone else is drinking:

_____
_____
_____
_____
_____
_____
_____

This is what I will say when people ask why I'm not drinking:

_____
_____
_____
_____
_____
_____
_____
_____

This is my plan to handle cravings:

_____
_____
_____
_____
_____
_____
_____
_____

(**Hint:** *Neurobiology of cravings, time-limited, know your triggers, take actions to ward off cravings*)

Here's how I plan to fill time previously spent drinking and address any chance of boredom or loneliness when not drinking:

___

___

___

___

___

___

___

___

(**Hint:** *Sports, outdoors, physical and exercise, arts and crafts, hobbies and other activities – like volunteering*)

(**Note:** *Depending upon the club and the social norms, you may need to anticipate and dodge or deal with drinking after the activity sessions. Forewarned is forearmed.*)

**Key to success:** Keep searching until you find something or some things that get you so excited and enthusiastic that it's what you want to spend every spare minute doing. When the desire to engage in this activity is so strong that it consumes your mind, endeavour to make it become your hobby – your new habit – above and beyond any unhealthy and damaging habit (or habits).

To manage insomnia or sleep issues after quitting alcohol, I will:

___

___

___

___

___

___

___

___

To manage relationships with people who still drink, I will:

_____
_____
_____
_____
_____
_____
_____
_____

These are some other issues and challenges I need to consider and manage:

_____
_____
_____
_____
_____
_____
_____
_____
_____

## Notes

_____
_____
_____
_____
_____
_____
_____
_____

# Chapter 6:

# Putting It Into Practice – Applying It to Your Life

## Overview

In the final chapter of your Companion Workbook, we turn theory into practice. This is where all the knowledge and insights you've gained come together to create a personalised, actionable plan for transforming your relationship with alcohol. The journey to this point has equipped you with a deep understanding of alcohol's effects and various strategies for quitting, and now it's time to apply that wisdom to your own life.

### *Why This Chapter Matters*

The final chapter is crucial because it bridges the gap between knowledge and action. It's one thing to understand the importance of quitting drinking or reducing your alcohol consumption, but implementing these changes in your daily life requires a structured approach and a clear plan. This chapter provides you with prompts, suggestions and resources to help you develop a step-by-step road map tailored to your unique needs and goals. By the end, you'll have a practical plan that you can start implementing immediately, empowering you to take control of your drinking decisions and create a brighter, healthier future.

## Reading Assignment, Chapter 6

Read Chapter 6 of *Ways to Quit Drinking: A Sober Curious Book on How to Control Alcohol for Better Health, Self-Esteem and Mental Clarity.*

Note down anything you want to take action on, or anything you feel the need to explore later – that's what will get the results for you, once you've crafted your implementation plan in the next steps.

## Summary Points from Chapter 6 of *Ways to Quit Drinking*

- **Create a personalised plan:** Utilise the information presented in earlier chapters and the knowledge you've gained to craft a detailed, step-by-step road map for achieving control over your relationship with alcohol and your drinking decisions.

- **Daily rituals for success:** Establish new, healthy daily rituals to replace your old habits. This includes morning and evening rituals that focus on mindfulness, gratitude and self-care as well as a health plan or a healthy life ritual to sharpen your focus on what to do.

- **Clarify your 'why':** Revisit and reinforce your reasons for wanting to change your relationship with alcohol. A strong, clear motivation is crucial for long-term success.

- **Manage long-term decisions:** Develop strategies to manage your decision to cut back or quit drinking over the long term. This includes exploring and noting down ideas for overcoming potential challenges and maintaining your new lifestyle. Be proactive, not reactive.

- **Address and release past issues:** Reflect on factors contributing to your relationship with alcohol and let go of any associated shame or self-blame. Acknowledge these factors and release them to move forward with compassion for yourself. This will likely involve working with a coach, counsellor or therapist or, at the very least, undertaking some self-help personal development.

- **Tailor your approach:** Choose and commit to the quit-drinking approaches that resonate with you and align with your values – for example, AA, MAT or the holistic approach. Customise your plan to fit your unique circumstances and preferences. Also think about who the supporters on your team will be.

- **Seek professional guidance:** Decide whether to work with a coach, therapist or other professionals to guide you through the emotional healing process. Their support can be invaluable for navigating the challenges of quitting or reducing alcohol consumption.

- **Prepare for social situations:** Develop responses and strategies for handling social situations where alcohol is present; this will reduce your fear of missing out (FOMO) and ensure you stay committed to your goals.

- **Overcome doubts and resistance:** Identify and address any lingering doubts or resistance to change, ensuring that your commitment to quitting or reducing alcohol consumption remains strong.

- **Celebrate your progress:** Acknowledge and celebrate each step forward, no matter how small, and adjust your plan as needed to stay on track towards a healthier, alcohol-free life.

## Purpose of Workbook Chapter 6

When you are finished with Workbook Chapter 6, you will have:

- **Crafted a personalised, step-by-step plan** to take control of your drinking decisions.

- **Established daily rituals** that promote mindfulness, gratitude and self-care, helping you build new, healthy habits.

- **Clarified your 'why'** for changing your relationship with alcohol, ensuring your motivation remains strong.

- **Developed strategies** to manage your decision over the long term, including ideas for overcoming challenges and maintaining your new lifestyle.

- **Reflected on and released past issues** related to your alcohol consumption, freeing yourself from shame and self-blame.

- **Chosen and committed to one or more quit-drinking approaches** that resonate with your values and circumstances.

- **Decided whether to work with a coach, therapist or other professional** to guide your emotional healing process, recognising the value of their support.

- **Prepared responses and strategies** for social situations involving alcohol, minimising FOMO and reinforcing your commitment to change.

- **Started to address and overcome any doubts or resistance** around your decision to quit or reduce your alcohol consumption, ensuring your commitment remains steadfast.

- **Celebrated your determination to achieve your better future and made a note to celebrate your progress** and adjust your plan as needed, staying on track toward a healthier, alcohol-free life.

*(**Tip:** Treat this as a 'living document', meaning it's not set in stone after you've written it down for the first time. This is just the starting point. Revisit the plan regularly. Choose a set time period – weekly, fortnightly, monthly – and adjust your plan as you find what works and what doesn't.)*

## Exercises for Chapter 6

### *Exercise 1: Action Plan – Template One*

Today's date: _____

My 'why':

_____
_____
_____
_____

My decision:

_____
_____
_____
_____

My personal goals:

_____
_____
_____
_____

My morning ritual:

_____
_____
_____
_____

My bedtime ritual:

_____
_____
_____
_____

My healthy life ritual:

_____
_____
_____
_____

These are the hobbies, activities and pastimes I am immersing myself in to determine if they're a long-term love for me or something I am doing just for now:

_____
_____
_____
_____
_____

Ways of quitting drinking I will adopt and pursue:

_____
_____
_____
_____
_____
_____
_____
_____

I will actively avoid these temptations, distractions and detrimental influences:

_____
_____
_____
_____
_____
_____
_____
_____

Reliable people I can contact when I need reassurance and support:

_____
_____
_____
_____
_____
_____
_____
_____

My non-alcoholic drinks of choice are:

At the time of day I would have previously been drinking alcohol, I now:

At social occasions when everyone else is drinking, I:

When people ask why I'm not drinking, I say:

_____
_____
_____
_____
_____
_____
_____

I handle cravings by:

_____
_____
_____
_____
_____
_____
_____

To fill time previously spent drinking and to address any chance of boredom or loneliness when not drinking, I fill my life and my soul with:

_____
_____
_____
_____
_____
_____
_____

I manage insomnia or sleep issues after quitting alcohol by:

_____
_____
_____
_____
_____
_____
_____
_____

I manage relationships with people who still drink by:

_____
_____
_____
_____
_____
_____
_____
_____

I am mindful of these other issues and challenges that I need to manage:

_____
_____
_____
_____
_____
_____
_____
_____

*Example: Action Plan – Template One*

**Today's date:** 20 June 2024

**My 'why':** I want to live a long, vibrant and healthy life.

**My decision:** I live an alcohol-free life

**My personal goals:** To show my friends and children that it's possible to be the 'life of the party' without alcohol.

**My morning ritual:** 5 deep breaths | 5 min meditation | stretching | glass of water with squeeze of lemon

**My bedtime ritual:** Turn off screens as early as possible | Eat dinner as early as possible | Lights out at a regular time

**My healthy life ritual:** Exercise daily (goal of 10,000 steps) | Maximum of 1 coffee per day | Avoid processed sugar | Drink 8 glasses of water

**These are the hobbies, activities and pastimes I am immersing myself in to determine if they're a long-term love for me or something I am doing just for now:**

I Loooove: Hiking | Keeping chickens | Renovating | Sewing

No spare time for anything else right now!

**Ways of quitting drinking I will adopt and pursue:**

Holistic approach – back to basics of nutritious diet (minimal to no processed foods); optimal sleep; active lifestyle – move a lot – minimum 10,000 steps to ward off low moods; learn self-development topics to understand how the human body works best (to the best of our current knowledge); meditate/calm my mind; manage my thoughts.

Coach – maintain regular sessions with my personal coach to address issues that stand in the way of achieving what I want.

**I actively avoid these temptations, distractions and detrimental influences:**

I acknowledge that the image of a glass of cold, dry white wine stirs a desire in me, so I keep in the forefront of my mind that the draw of the image and the desire is more appealing than how I will feel after indulging in it.

**Reliable people I can contact when I need reassurance and support:**

My coach

Like-minded people in Facebook groups for those aspiring to be alcohol free

**My non-alcoholic drinks of choice are:**

Mineral water with a squeeze of lemon or lime juice. Mineral water with elderflower cordial.

Lemon lime and bitters when out.

**At the time of day I would have previously been drinking alcohol, I now:**

Drink mineral water with a squeeze of lemon or lime juice. I walk the dog. I get laundry put away to keep a tidy house. I plan my following day.

**At social occasions when everyone else is drinking, I:**

Feel special. I feel strong and powerful. I feel cosy in myself that I have no ethyl alcohol in my bloodstream to challenge my health. I draw on the knowledge that I have spent time learning about my values, who I am, what legacy I want to leave and what I want to fit into my life, and I feel content being in the moment with a focus on observing, enjoying and immersing myself in the event or occasion I am at to absorb it, to grow from the experience and to interact with others around me and connect in the way humans can. If it's a poor environment, with a negative culture or seedy undertones, I plan my earliest possible escape!

**When people ask why I'm not drinking, I say:**

I don't enjoy it anymore.

I'm prioritising my health.

**I handle cravings by:**

Remembering how totally rotten and disgusted with myself I feel when alcohol becomes the one in control…

**To fill time previously spent drinking and to address any chance of boredom or loneliness when not drinking, I fill my life and my soul with:**

I have my glass of mineral water with a squeeze of lemon or lime juice close to hand. I connect with my family and pets. I keep busy – I keep my house and affairs and the like in order. I plan for fun activities and projects and occasions so there is never a chance for boredom. If I need to keep my hands occupied, I garden or do jigsaws or crochet.

**I manage insomnia or sleep issues after quitting alcohol by:**

Educating myself about the fascinating 'science of sleep' and how it underpins health, and learning what the science says about how to optimise it. I wear a smart watch to understand my sleep patterns and try to work out what negatively affects the quality of my sleep. If it all goes pear-shaped, I seek medical advice.

**I manage relationships with people who still drink by:**

If they are a true friend, who respects me and my choice, they don't 'give me a hard time' about not drinking, just as I don't criticise their decision to drink alcohol. So, I spend time alongside other people to enjoy them for who they are, and allow them the choices they make. If the interaction is uncomfortable, unpleasant, negative or otherwise not to my liking, I extract myself as quickly and thoroughly as possible. This had to start with me gaining my own self-confidence and self-respect.

**I am mindful of these other issues and challenges to manage:**

There are times when I feel a pang that I can't have that glass of white wine. I bring to mind the enhanced quality of life and clarity of mind and greater success I have experienced ever since becoming alcohol free.

One day I may travel again, and if I find myself in a Scottish pub with whiskey in my nostrils or stout beer frothing in front of me, I know I will be challenged. They weren't my 'poison', but they were experiences I once or twice enjoyed about alcohol. Would I be tempted? Would I still be worthy of being the author of a book about *Ways to Quit Drinking* if I weakened? Would I weaken? Right now, I choose not to worry about this, as it may never happen. If I find myself in that situation in the future, I think I will enjoy the aroma, perhaps dip a finger in the whiskey (and hope I don't get caught by whoever's drink it is?) for the burn, and leave it be. It's simply not worth it to go backwards. And I know it's a slippery slope…

## Exercise 2: Action Plan – Template Two

| | | |
|---|---|---|
| My Personal GOALS | **MY BEST LIFE**<br><br>Today's Date | Morning Ritual |
| Healthy Life Ritual | | My Supporters |
| | **My "WHY"** | |
| In Response to "You're Not Drinking?" I say: | | Bedtime Ritual |
| Hobbies & Habits to Fulfill & Bring Joy | My Alcohol-Free Beverage Options | I Will Avoid: |

*Example: Action Plan – Template Two*

**My Personal GOALS**
Show my friends & family that it is possible to be the "life of the party" without alcohol.

**MY BEST LIFE**
Today's Date
20 June 2024

**Morning Ritual**
5 Deep Breaths
Stretching
5 mins Meditation
Glass of Water w. a dash of Apple Cider Vinegar.

**Healthy Life Ritual**
– Daily –
Walk 30+ minutes
Maximum 1 coffee
Avoid sugar
Avoid processed foods
Drink 8 glasses water.

**My "WHY"**
I want to live a long and healthy life with vibrancy.

**My Supporters**
My Coach
My Walking Group
My Wholistic Wellbeing Health Advisor

**In Response to "You're Not Drinking?" I say:**
"I don't enjoy it"

**Bedtime Ritual**
Turn OFF screens as early as possible.
Regular bedtime.
Evening meal early.

**Hobbies & Habits to Fulfill & Bring Joy**
Hiking
Keeping Chickens
Sewing
Renovating

**My Alcohol-Free Beverage Options**
Mineral water w. a squeeze of lime juice.
Lemon, lime and bitters when out.

**I Will Avoid:**
Thoughts that alcohol has any benefits.
Thoughts that I am missing out on anything.

# Keys to Success

Making a major lifestyle change like this is no small feat. To stay committed and motivated, keep these three things in mind:

1. Always remember your 'why':

    o Keep your reasons for quitting front and centre.

    o Write them down and refer to them often, especially when temptation threatens to strike.

2. Fully embrace the benefits of your new lifestyle:

    o Celebrate your clear head, improved sleep, increased energy and enhanced presence.

    o Appreciate how much easier it is to work towards your goals without alcohol holding you back.

3. When an urge arises, play the tape forward:

    o Allow yourself to briefly remember the worst parts of drinking – the hangovers, the shame, the lost time.

    o Contrast that with all you've gained from adopting an alcohol-free lifestyle.

Define what success looks like for you and keep that vision in mind. Whether it's improved relationships, better health, career progression or personal growth, keeping your 'eyes on the prize' will help you stay the course.

## *Notes*

_____
_____
_____
_____
_____
_____

Dear Reader,

Thank you for choosing and reading our WAYS TO QUIT DRINKING – COMPANION WORKBOOK. We hope this book has provided you with valuable insights and practical tips that you can apply in your life. Your feedback is incredibly important, as it helps us continue to improve and provide valuable content to readers like you.

If you found this book helpful and enjoyable, we'd be most grateful if you could please take a moment to leave a positive review on Amazon. Your constructive feedback and max-star rating would mean the world to us! And would help others discover and benefit from this Companion Workbook as well.

You can leave your review by clicking this link: Your Opinion Matters

or scanning the QR code below:

If you have any comments, feedback or suggestions for improvement, we would love to hear from you. Please feel free to reach out to us at feedback@organisedcoaching.com .

Thank you once again for your support and for being a valued reader.

Warmest regards,

Michelle Matthews and Tony Matthews

Wrap-Up:

# Your Journey Towards Better Health, Self-Esteem and Mental Clarity

Congratulations on completing this Companion Workbook to *Ways to Quit Drinking*! You've taken a significant step towards transforming your relationship with alcohol and reclaiming control over your life. As you reflect on your journey so far, remember that this workbook is designed to evolve with you. It's not just a set of instructions but a dynamic tool for personal growth and discovery.

## Embracing Your Exciting Future

Your commitment to this process is admirable. By creating a personalised plan and exploring new strategies for self-care and fulfilment, you've set a course for a brighter future. As you continue forward, keep these key points in mind:

- **A living document:** Your plan is not set in stone. Embrace the flexibility to adjust and refine your strategies as you learn and grow.

- **Regular reflection:** Schedule regular check-ins – weekly, fortnightly or monthly – to assess your progress, celebrate your achievements and adjust your course as needed.

- **Seeking support:** Healing your inner self is crucial to breaking free from alcohol dependence. Lean on trusted coaches, counsellors or support groups to help you navigate challenges and maintain your motivation.

## Nurturing Self-Care and Healing

Healing your 'insides' is a vital aspect of this exercise. Here are some self-care practices to consider:

- **Mindfulness and meditation:** These practices can help you stay present and manage stress effectively. Explore some yoga classes to find a peace-filled instructor who instils a sense of wellbeing and calm in you when you attend their classes.

- **Physical wellbeing:** Prioritise regular exercise, healthy eating and adequate sleep to support your overall health and wellbeing. Seriously – this is non-negotiable.

- **Emotional support:** Take whatever steps you can to build a strong support network of friends, family and peers who understand and encourage your journey.

## Celebrating Your Progress

Celebrate every milestone, no matter how small. Each step forward is a testament to your strength and determination. Remember, setbacks are a natural part of change. Be patient and compassionate with yourself as you navigate this new phase of your life.

## Looking Ahead

As you close this chapter and move forward, remember that your path towards freedom from alcohol is a path towards a life of greater joy, purpose and fulfilment. Stay curious, embrace new experiences and never lose sight of your ultimate goal – a life free from alcohol's grip.

## Final Thoughts

Your decision to prioritise your wellbeing is a powerful one. By investing in yourself and your future, you're creating a life that aligns with your values and aspirations. Trust in your ability to make lasting change and know that you are never alone on this path.

Thank you for allowing us to be a part of your journey. Here's to your courage, your resilience and the extraordinary life you're creating – one day at a time.

# Appendix

Please see below the answers to the questions in Chapter 1.

## Fill in the Blanks – Industrial Applications

1. Ethanol and isopropanol
2. Preservation
3. Freezing
4. Fossil
5. Ethanol and ethanol

## Multiple Choice Quiz – Lesser-Known Health Impacts

1. C: International Agency for Research on Cancer (IARC)
2. C: Alcohol consumption increases breast cancer risk
3. B: Pancreatic cancer
4. C: Liver disease
5. C: It can elevate blood pressure and disrupt heart rhythm
6. C: Chronic heavy drinking can lead to cognitive impairment and memory loss
7. B: Tooth decay
8. C: By drying out the mouth and promoting bacterial growth
9. C: It suppresses REM sleep
10. B: It is essential for memory consolidation and learning

11. C: By disrupting the brain's process of clearing out harmful toxins

12. C: Higher risk of cognitive development issues

13. D: To safeguard foetal health

14. B: Mindful observation and consideration of alcohol's effects are encouraged

15. D: To assess how alcohol affects yourself

# References

Abrahao, K. P., Salinas, A. G., & Lovinger, D. M. (2017). Alcohol and the brain: Neuronal molecular targets, synapses, and circuits. *Neuron, 96*(6), 1223–1238. https://doi.org/10.1016/j.neuron.2017.10.032

Adriaanse, M. A., Gollwitzer, P. M., De Ridder, D. T. D., de Wit, J. B. F., & Kroese, F. M. (2011). Breaking habits with implementation intentions: A test of underlying processes. *Personality and Social Psychology Bulletin, 37*(4), 502–513. https://doi.org/10.1177/0146167211399102

Afifi, T. O., Enns, M. W., Cox, B. J., Asmundson, G. J., Stein, M. B., & Sareen, J. (2008). Population attributable fractions of psychiatric disorders and suicide ideation and tries associated with adverse childhood experiences. *American Journal of Public Health, 98*(5), 946-952. https://doi.org/10.2105/AJPH.2007.120253

Audiffren, M., André, N., & Baumeister, R. F. (2022). Training willpower: Reducing costs and valuing effort. *Frontiers in Neuroscience, 16*. https://doi.org/10.3389/fnins.2022.699817

Ayyar, A. (2019, June 7). The ultimate guide to Ramana Maharshi's self-inquiry. *Sifting to the Truth.* https://www.siftingtothetruth.com/blog/2019/6/7/the-ultimate-guide-to-spiritual-self-inquiry

Becker, H. C. (2012). Effects of alcohol dependence and withdrawal on stress responsiveness and alcohol consumption. *Alcohol Research: Current Reviews, 34*(4), 448–458. https://www.ncbi.nlm.nih.gov/pmc/articles/PMC3860383/

Brady, K. T., & Back, S. E. (2012). Childhood trauma, posttraumatic stress disorder, and alcohol dependence. *Alcohol Research: Current Reviews, 34*(4), 408–413. https://www.ncbi.nlm.nih.gov/pmc/articles/PMC3860395/

Burri, A., Maercker, A., Krammer, S., & Simmen-Janevska, K. (2013). Childhood trauma and PTSD symptoms increase the risk of cognitive impairment in a sample of former indentured child laborers in old age. *PLoS ONE, 8*(2), e57826. https://doi.org/10.1371/journal.pone.0057826

Carrigan, M. A., Uryasev, O., Frye, C. B., Eckman, B. L., Myers, C. R., Hurley, T. D., & Benner, S. A. (2014). Hominids adapted to metabolize ethanol long before human-directed fermentation. *Proceedings of the National Academy of Sciences, 112*(2), 458–463. https://doi.org/10.1073/pnas.1404167111

Chiva-Blanch, G., & Badimon, L. (2019). Benefits and risks of moderate alcohol consumption on cardiovascular disease: Current findings and controversies. *Nutrients*, 12(1), 108. https://doi.org/10.3390/nu12010108

Church, D., Stapleton, P., Mollon, P., Feinstein, D., Boath, E., Mackay, D., & Sims, R. (2018). Guidelines for the treatment of PTSD using clinical EFT (emotional freedom techniques). *Healthcare*, 6(4). https://doi.org/10.3390/healthcare6040146

Colrain, I. M., Nicholas, C. L., & Baker, F. C. (2014). Alcohol and the sleeping brain. In E. V. Sullivan & A. Pfefferbaum (Eds.), *Handbook of Clinical Neurology*, *125*, 415–431. https://doi.org/10.1016/B978-0-444-62619-6.00024-0

Daniel, T. O., Stanton, C. M., & Epstein, L. H. (2013). The future is now: Reducing impulsivity and energy intake using episodic future thinking. *Psychological Science*, 24(11), 2339–2342. https://doi.org/10.1177/0956797613488780

Edenberg, H. (2013). Genetics of alcohol use disorders. In P. M. Miller (Ed.), *biological research on addiction: Comprehensive addictive behaviors and disorders*, Volume 2. Elsevier. https://doi.org/10.1016/C2011-0-07782-7

Elhai, J. D., Levine, J. C., Dvorak, R. D., & Hall, B. J. (2016). Fear of missing out, need for touch, anxiety and depression are related to problematic smartphone use. *Computers in Human Behavior*, 63, 509-516. https://psycnet.apa.org/doi/10.1016/j.chb.2016.05.079

Gardner, B., Lally, P., & Wardle, J. (2012). Making health habitual: The psychology of 'habit-formation' and general practice. *British Journal of General Practice*, *62*(605), 664–666. https://doi.org/10.3399/bjgp12X659466

Grant, A. M., Franklin, J., & Langford, P. (2002). The self-reflection and insight scale: A new measure of private self-consciousness. *Social Behavior and Personality*, *30*(8), 821-836. http://dx.doi.org/10.1177/0306422010390622

Greenberg, L. S. (2017). *Emotion-focused therapy*. American Psychological Association. https://doi.org/10.1037/15971-001

Higuchi, S., Matsushita, S., Muramatsu, T., Murayama, M., & Hayashida, M. (1996). Alcohol and aldehyde dehydrogenase genotypes and drinking behavior in Japanese. *Alcoholism: Clinical and Experimental Research*, *20*(3), 493–497. https://doi.org/10.1111/j.1530-0277.1996.tb01080.x

Hoyumpa, A. M. (1986). Mechanisms of vitamin deficiencies in alcoholism. *Alcoholism: Clinical and Experimental Research*, *10*(6), 573–581. https://doi.org/10.1111/j.1530-0277.1986.tb05147.x

Jemberie, W. B., Padyab, M., Snellman, F., & Lundgren, L. (2020). A multidimensional latent class analysis of harmful alcohol use among older adults: Subtypes within the Swedish Addiction Severity Index Registry. *Journal of Addiction Medicine*, *14*(4), e89–e99. https://doi.org/10.1097/adm.0000000000000636

Kesmodel, U., Wisborg, K., Olsen, S. F., Henriksen, T. B., & Secher, N. J. (2002). Moderate alcohol intake in pregnancy and the risk of spontaneous abortion. *Alcohol and Alcoholism*, *37*(1), 87–92. https://doi.org/10.1093/alcalc/37.1.87

Kono, S., Ikeda, M., Tokudome, S., Nishizumi, M., & Kuratsune, M. (1986). Alcohol and mortality: A cohort study of male Japanese physicians. *International Journal of Epidemiology*, *15*(4), 527–532. https://doi.org/10.1093/ije/15.4.527

Kushner, M. G., Abrams, K., Thuras, P., Hanson, K. L., Brekke, M., & Sletten, S. (2005). Follow-up study of anxiety disorder and alcohol dependence in comorbid alcoholism treatment patients. *Alcoholism: Clinical & Experimental Research*, *29*(8), 1432–1443. https://doi.org/10.1097/01.alc.0000175072.17623.f8

Lookatch, S. J., Wimberly, A. S., & McKay, J. R. (2019). Effects of social support and 12-step involvement on recovery among people in continuing care for cocaine dependence. *Substance Use & Misuse*, *54*(13), 2144–2155. https://doi.org/10.1080/10826084.2019.1638406

Maraboli, S. (2022, January 2). *Incredible change happens in your life when you decide to take control of what you do have power over instead of craving control over what you don't* [Image attached] [Status update]. Facebook. https://www.facebook.com/photo/?fbid=2821065447916136&set=a.690866084269427

McDonald, J. A., Goyal, A., & Terry, M. B. (2013). Alcohol intake and breast cancer risk: Weighing the overall evidence. *Current Breast Cancer Reports*, *5*(3), 208–221. https://doi.org/10.1007/s12609-013-0114-z

Mehta, D., Klengel, T., Conneely, K. N., Smith, A. K., Altmann, A., Pace, T. W., Rex-Haffner, M., Loeschner, A., Gonik, M., Mercer, K. B., Bradley, B., Muller-Myhsok, B., Ressler, K. J., & Binder, E. B. (2013). Childhood maltreatment is associated with distinct genomic and epigenetic profiles in posttraumatic stress disorder. *Proceedings of the National Academy of Sciences*, *110*(20), 8302–8307. https://doi.org/10.1073/pnas.1217750110

Mercille, J. (2017). Media coverage of alcohol issues: A critical political economy framework—A case study from Ireland. *International Journal of Environmental Research and Public Health*, *14*(6), 650. https://doi.org/10.3390/ijerph14060650

Merikangas, K. R., Stevens, D., & Fenton, B. (1996). Comorbidity of alcoholism and anxiety disorders: The role of family studies. *Alcohol Health and Research World, 20*(2), 100–106. https://www.ncbi.nlm.nih.gov/pmc/articles/PMC6876502/

Miller, W. R., Walters, S. T., & Bennett, M. E. (2001). How effective is alcoholism treatment in the United States? *Journal of Studies on Alcohol, 62*(2), 211–220. https://doi.org/10.15288/jsa.2001.62.211

Moos, R. H., & Moos, B. S. (2006). Participation in treatment and Alcoholics Anonymous: A 16-year follow-up of initially untreated individuals. *Journal of Clinical Psychology, 62*(6), 735–750. https://doi.org/10.1002/jclp.20259

Nemeroff, C. B. (2003). The role of GABA in the pathophysiology and treatment of anxiety disorders. *Psychopharmacology Bulletin, 37*(4), 133–146.

Nestor, J. (2020). *Breath: the new science of a lost art.* Riverhead Books.

NPR Staff. (2014, March 24). *With sobering science, doctor debunks 12-step recovery.* NPR. https://www.npr.org/2014/03/23/291405829/with-sobering-science-doctor-debunks-12-step-recovery

Oberst, U., Wegmann, E., Stodt, B., Brand, M., & Chamarro, A. (2017). Negative consequences from heavy social networking in adolescents: The mediating role of fear of missing out. *Journal of Adolescence, 55*, 51-60. https://doi.org/10.1016/j.adolescence.2016.12.00

Oh, V. K. S., Sarwar, A., & Pervez, N. (2022). The study of mindfulness as an intervening factor for enhanced psychological well-being in building the level of resilience. *Frontiers in Psychology, 13.* https://doi.org/10.3389/fpsyg.2022.1056834

O'Leary, C. M., Taylor, C., Zubrick, S. R., Kurinczuk, J. J., & Bower, C. (2013). Prenatal alcohol exposure and educational achievement in children aged 8-9 years. *Pediatrics, 132*(2), e468-475. https://doi.org/10.1542/peds.2012-3002

Oppezzo, M., & Schwartz, D. L. (2014). Give your ideas some legs: The positive effects of walking on creative thinking. *Journal of Experimental Psychology: Learning, Memory, and Cognition, 40*(4), 1142–1152. http://dx.doi.org/10.1037/a0036577

Osna, N. A., Donohue, T. M., & Kharbanda, K. K. (2017). Alcoholic liver disease: Pathogenesis and current management. *Alcohol Research: Current Reviews, 38*(2), 147–161. https://www.ncbi.nlm.nih.gov/pmc/articles/PMC5513682/

Palzes, V. A., Parthasarathy, S., Chi, F. W., Kline-Simon, A. H., Lu, Y., Weisner, C., Ross, T. B., Elson, J., & Sterling, S. A. (2020). Associations between psychiatric disorders and alcohol consumption levels in an adult primary care population. *Alcoholism: Clinical and Experimental Research*, *44*(12), 2536–2544. https://doi.org/10.1111/acer.14477

Peppard, P. E., Austin, D., & Brown, R. L. (2007). Association of alcohol consumption and sleep disordered breathing in men and women. *Journal of Clinical Sleep Medicine*, *3*(3), 265–270. https://www.ncbi.nlm.nih.gov/pmc/articles/PMC2564771/265–270.

Petti, S., & Scully, C. (2005). Alcohol consumption and oral cancer: a study in Italy. *British Journal of Cancer*, *92*(5), 899–900.

Piano, M. R. (2017). Alcohol's effects on the cardiovascular system. *Alcohol Research: Current Reviews*, *38*(2), 219–241. https://www.ncbi.nlm.nih.gov/pmc/articles/PMC5513687/

Przybylski, A. K., Murayama, K., DeHaan, C. R., & Gladwell, V. (2013). Motivational, emotional, and behavioral correlates of fear of missing out. *Computers in Human Behavior*, *29*(4), 1841–1848https://doi.org/10.1016/j.chb.2013.02.014

Robertson, A. G., Easter, M. M., Lin, H., Frisman, L. K., Swanson, J. W., & Swartz, M. S. (2018). Medication-assisted treatment for alcohol-dependent adults with serious mental illness and criminal justice involvement: Effects on treatment utilization and outcomes. *American Journal of Psychiatry*, *175*(7), 665–673. https://doi.org/10.1176/appi.ajp.2018.17060688

Sabia, S., Elbaz, A., Britton, A., Bell, S., Dugravot, A., Shipley, M., Kivimaki, M., & Singh-Manoux, A. (2014). Alcohol consumption and cognitive decline in early old age. *Neurology*, *82*(4), 332–339. https://doi.org/10.1212/wnl.0000000000000063

Schuckit, M. A. (2009). An overview of genetic influences in alcoholism. *Journal of Substance Abuse Treatment*, *36*(1), S5–14. https://pubmed.ncbi.nlm.nih.gov/19062348/

Schuckit, M. A., Tipp, J. E., Reich, T., Hesselbrock, v. M., & Bucholz, K. K. (2006). The histories of withdrawal convulsions and delirium tremens in 1648 alcohol dependent subjects. *Addiction*, *90*(10), 1335–1347. https://doi.org/10.1046/j.1360-0443.1995.901013355.x

Scott, C., & Corbin, W. R. (2014). Influence of sensation seeking on response to alcohol versus placebo: Implications for the acquired preparedness model. *Journal of Studies on Alcohol and Drugs*, *75*(1), 136–144. https://doi.org/10.1046/j.1360-0443.1995.901013355.x

Shin, S. H., Hong, H. G., & Jeon, S.-M. (2012). Personality and alcohol use: The role of impulsivity. *Addictive Behaviors*, *37*(1), 102–107. https://doi.org/10.1016/j.addbeh.2011.09.006

Smith, R. J., & Laiks, L. S. (2018). Behavioral and neural mechanisms underlying habitual and compulsive drug seeking. *Progress in Neuro-Psychopharmacology and Biological Psychiatry*, *87*, 11–21. https://doi.org/10.1016/j.pnpbp.2017.09.003

Sood, B., Delaney-Black, V., Covington, C., Nordstrom-Klee, B., Ager, J., Templin, T., Janisse, J., Martier, S., & Sokol, R. J. (2001). Prenatal alcohol exposure and childhood behavior at age 6 to 7 years: I. Dose-response effect. *Pediatrics*, *108*(2), e34. https://doi.org/10.1542/peds.108.2.e34

Soundararajan, S., Narayanan, G., Agrawal, A., Prabhakaran, D., & Murthy, P. (2017). Relation between age at first alcohol drink & adult life drinking patterns in alcohol-dependent patients. *The Indian Journal of Medical Research*, *146*(5), 606–611. https://doi.org/10.4103%2Fijmr.IJMR_1363_15

Stockwell, T., Zhao, J., Panwar, S., Roemer, A., Naimi, T., & Chikritzhs, T. (2016). Do "moderate" drinkers have reduced mortality risk? A systematic review and meta-analysis of alcohol consumption and all-cause mortality. *Journal of Studies on Alcohol and Drugs*, *77*(2), 185–198. https://doi.org/10.15288/jsad.2016.77.185

Taillieu, T. L., Brownridge, D. A., Sareen, J., & Afifi, T. O. (2016). Childhood emotional maltreatment and mental disorders: Results from a nationally representative adult sample from the United States. *Child Abuse & Neglect*, *59*, 1–12. https://doi.org/10.1016/j.chiabu.2016.07.005

Testino, G. (2011). The burden of cancer attributable to alcohol consumption. *Maedica*, *6*(4), 313–320. https://www.ncbi.nlm.nih.gov/pmc/articles/PMC3391950/

Tezal, M., Grossi, S. G., Ho, A. W., & Genco, R. J. (2001). The effect of alcohol consumption on periodontal disease. *Journal of Periodontology*, 72(2), 183–189. https://doi.org/10.1902/jop.2001.72.2.183

Traversy, G., & Chaput, J.-P. (2018). Alcohol consumption and obesity: An update. *Current Obesity Reports*, *4*(1), 122–130. https://doi.org/10.1007%2Fs13679-014-0129-4

Tyas, S. L. (2001). Alcohol use and the risk of developing Alzheimer's disease. *Alcohol Research & Health*, *25*(4), 299–306. https://www.ncbi.nlm.nih.gov/pmc/articles/pmc6705707/

Wakabayashi, M., Sugiyama, Y., Takada, M., Kinjo, A., Iso, H., & Tabuchi, T. (2022). Loneliness and increased hazardous alcohol use: Data from a nationwide internet survey with 1-year follow-up. *International Journal of Environmental Research and Public Health*, *19*(19), 12086. https://doi.org/10.3390/ijerph191912086

Walker, M. P. (2017). *Why we sleep: Unlocking the power of sleep and dreams*. Scribner.

Xie, L., Kang, H., Xu, Q., Chen, M. J., Liao, Y., Thiyagarajan, M., O'Donnell, J., Christensen, D. J., Nicholson, C., Iliff, J. J., Takano, T., Deane, R., & Nedergaard, M. (2013). Sleep drives metabolite clearance from the adult brain. *Science*, *342*(6156), 373-7.

Zhang, C., Qing, N., & Zhang, S. (2021). The impact of leisure activities on the mental health of older adults: The mediating effect of social support and perceived stress. *Journal of Healthcare Engineering*, 2021, 6264447. https://doi.org/10.1155/2021/6264447

Made in the USA
Las Vegas, NV
10 August 2024

93647321R00063